QUEER AGING

QUEER AGING

The Gayby Boomers and a New Frontier for Gerontology

JESUS RAMIREZ-VALLES

OXFORD
UNIVERSITY PRESS

OXFORD
UNIVERSITY PRESS

Oxford University Press is a department of the University of Oxford. It furthers the University's objective of excellence in research, scholarship, and education by publishing worldwide. Oxford is a registered trade mark of Oxford University Press in the UK and certain other countries.

Published in the United States of America by Oxford University Press
198 Madison Avenue, New York, NY 10016, United States of America.

Library of Congress Cataloging-in-Publication Data
Names: Ramirez-Valles, Jesus, author.
Title: Queer Aging: The Gayby Boomers and a New Frontier for Gerontology / Jesus Ramirez-Valles.
Description: 1 Edition. | New York : Oxford University Press, 2016.
Identifiers: LCCN 2016000960 (print) | LCCN 2016023003 (ebook) |
ISBN 9780190276348 (paperback) | ISBN 9780190276355 (UPDF) |
ISBN 9780190276362 (EPUB) | ISBN 9780190276379 (Online Component)
Subjects: LCSH: Older gays. | Aging—Social aspects. | Older gays—Care. |
BISAC: MEDICAL / Public Health. | MEDICAL / Geriatrics. | SOCIAL SCIENCE / Gay Studies.
Classification: LCC HQ76.27.O44 R36 2016 (print) | LCC HQ76.27.O44 (ebook) |
DDC 306.76/60846—dc23
LC record available at https://lccn.loc.gov/2016000960

9 8 7 6 5 4 3 2

Printed by Webcom, Inc., Canada

For Brad and Cameron and the life we create

CONTENTS

PREFACE

> I became obsessed with age. At 17, I dreaded growing old.
>
> Old age is something that must never happen to me.
>
> The image of myself in the mirror must never fade into someone I cant (sic) look at.
>
> —RECHY, *2013 [1963], p. 66*

I'm not a gerontologist. As a matter of fact, I was not interested in old age, perhaps because of my belief in my eternal youth. I'm gay, yet not "older"—as in 55 or older. I come to the study of aging and queerness through my life's work in public health, particularly in HIV/AIDS with gay and bisexual men and transgender women. I came out as a gay man in the midst of the epidemic in México. I started exploring the gay scene in 1985 in México, with no consciousness of AIDS or aging. A few years later, I found myself organizing communities of gay men and picking up and burying the bodies of those who succumbed to AIDS. I have studied AIDS and the experiences of gay men. In that time, I witnessed the transformation of the gay person from scarcely being in an emaciated body, with sunken, pale cheeks, to being in an energized, athletic, muscular, manly figure on preexposure prophylaxis. I belong to the generation marked by AIDS.

I have always been around older gay men, but I was not conscious of the social and cultural implications of age until the early 2000s. In my 20s I was surrounded by gay men who were 15 to 20 years older than me—guys who would fall under the category of "older gay men." My darling friend Oscar was in his late 40s when we were organizing and educating gay men in Juárez, México. Marcos was the third in this threesome of AIDS activists, and I still refer to him respectfully and amorously as our "mother." Others, not so kindly, called him *abuela* (grandmother). Oscar himself used the term in a self-deprecating manner, so I thought, but I had not grasped the phenomenon of older age.

My first partner, during the 1990s, was 17 years my senior and, although we separated many years ago, I have witnessed his aging: retirement, a couple of heart surgeries, painful arthritis, caring for his dying parents and siblings, rejecting the idea of living in a retirement community in a warmer climate, and turning a deaf ear to his doctor's insistence to quit smoking.

Three years ago, another friend, Carlos (not his real name), killed himself at the age of 64 in California. "They say he died of sadness," a mutual friend wrote on Facebook the morning we learned of his death. Carlos lived with HIV for 25 years. He left Cuba during the Mariel boatlift, fleeing the "macho" revolution. In the same group of refugees was Reinaldo Arenas, one of the most prolific and fervent Cuban writers of the second half of the 20th century. Arenas, a gay man, also suffered from AIDS and committed suicide in 1990 in Manhattan. He was 47 years old. And, like my friend Carlos, he had married and had children during his younger years in Cuba.

My friend Carlos fought AIDS, exile, homophobia, and melancholia. He battled HIV and AIDS long enough to benefit from antiretroviral therapy. He aged with HIV and the seemingly perpetual sadness. Carlos was able to build a very successful, professional career in the United States, thanks largely to antiretroviral therapy. Wise, smart, witty, and handsome, he always had friends and men who loved him. He even competed in Track and Field in the Olympic Gay Games. Many of us never saw the other side—his depression. His surviving partner of 10 years, Matt, however, knew of that inner anguish very well. He toured the country with Carlos in search of treatment, clinics, and psychiatrists that could relieve his depression. So many times Matt rushed home or to a clinic after a phone call telling him Carlos had made yet another suicide attempt. Carlos' passing came to me as a reminder of AIDS—gay men dying during the 1980s and early part of the 1990s—in a time when we now think of HIV as a "manageable" chronic condition. His friendship drew me close to the experience of aging, aging as a gay person and with HIV. Men of his generation are unique, yet unnoticed in the field of gerontology.

So, when confronted with the question of what my next project should be, after years of doing research on HIV with gay men, the subject of aging was the answer. This task is an instinctive progression of my work and my own experience tracking the epidemic of AIDS, directing my attention to the lives of older gay men. With this project I also wished to overcome the limitations of my previous research with gay men. Despite my own will, I had been boxed in as the "Latino" researcher. This racist academic practice and my own consciousness about it prevented me from delving into the larger gay male experience (from a scholarly point of view). I decided that, for *Queer Aging*, I would expand my own understanding by including what we call, in our shorthand racial discourse, white and black older gay men. The benefit of doing this is the analysis of commonalities and differences as well as the layered systems of race and sexuality (besides that of HIV status and social class position) in old age—what some scholars call *intersectionality*.

My second limitation was that I ignored the effects of age, history, and cohort—that is, the life course—in the lives of gay men. I treated all men in the samples I studied as equally affected by age, historical events, and cohort culture. This is not only my shortcoming, but one of many scholars as well. One reason behind this limitation is the infancy of our field and the restricted tools we have. The most we have been able to do is to "control" for age or focus on traditionally defined areas, such as childhood development (but not aging). As I write this, I am collaborating tangentially with colleagues who are beginning to apply the life course perspective empirically to understand the experiences of sexual minorities. In this book, then, I examine a group of gay men who have aged together facing similar experiences and sociopolitical forces, and who (perhaps) share a culture. In *Queer Aging*, I look at the experiences of older sexual minorities as shaped by their own age, their cohort, and the history that accompanies them.

Another impetus for the timing of this project is the maturing of the Baby Boomers. In 2011, the midst of my fieldwork for this book, the oldest members of the Baby Boomer generation turned 65 and in, 2014, the youngest became 50. This was heralded as a major milestone that would change the aging experience in the United States (Rowley, 2012). The unprecedented large size of this cohort puts new demands on our health and social services and pension systems. The unique cultural outlook of this group—very different from the preceding Silent Generation (born between 1925 and 1945)—also signals changes in the aging experience, from living arrangements and work to expectations about sexuality and body image. Even more important is the Baby Boomer generation came of age during the gay liberation movement, creating the first cohort of openly lesbian, gay, bisexual, and transgender (LGBT) people.

For these reasons, I believe it to be a crucial time to examine the experiences of gay men of the Baby Boomer generation. They are the first to age identifying as "gay men," they are the hardest hit by the AIDS epidemic, and now they are counted in the largest group of aging people—many aging with HIV. My starting question was: What is it like to be an older gay man? From this query I derived more specific questions: How do gay men experience old age? How does race mold such experience? How does HIV, if at all, make a difference in aging?

I turned to my gerontology colleagues for help. They offered guidance to the central concerns of aging (or gerontology) research: life transitions, chronic illness and comorbidity, social support, independent living, and successful aging. I then began to take stock of the existing research on older gay men. At the same time, I started hanging out with various groups of older LGBT individuals, most of them in social services agencies in Chicago. I conducted one-on-one in-depth interviews and group discussions with older gay men. I published my first scholarly article in the discipline (Ramirez-Valles, Dirkes, Berrett, 2014). In it, I explored the influences of social support on mental health in a sample of older gay men. This book emerges from all that work.

I quickly realized that gerontology is a very conservative field—a view confirmed by colleagues working with older queer folks. Early during this project, I contacted a leading research center that was undertaking its first study on sexuality in older age using a national representative sample of community dwellers. Investigators were gathering not only traditional data on health, sexual practices, and income and education, but also they were doing physical examinations and collecting biospecimens. My query was about gender and sexual orientation: Do you have data on participants' gender and sexual orientation identity? "No," was the response I received. When asked why not, I was told, "Those types of questions are very intrusive." (This was in 2010!) At that moment, I lost my ability to articulate a logical counterargument, which often happens when speaking to a customer service representative.

Gerontology, in its current form, is unable (and somewhat unwilling) to capture the experiences of gay men (and other sexual minorities, for sure). It actually silences and distorts their voices. Gerontology is largely an empirical enterprise, devoid of critical discussions of concepts and theories, except for a few scholars working from Marxist and feminist perspectives. The empirical drive is dangerous because it hides the observer's subjectivity and taken-for-granted world (e.g., heterosexual and white). It pretends to be objective when we—queer people of color, and scholars—know very well there is no objective science.

I then decided to put on the lenses of sexuality and queer studies to counter the prevalent gerontology agenda and read the experiences of gay men's aging. Queer research, it turns out, was not doing much either. It barely speaks about old bodies. I found only a handful of scholars writing on the subject, and I'm indebted to them for their thinking, which contributes to the foundation to this book. In *Queer Aging*, I place these two perspectives, gerontology and queer/sexuality studies, in dialogue to read and interpret the narratives of gay men.

This project would have not been possible without the men who shared their stories with me. I genuinely appreciate their kindness and sincerity. I also benefited from the wisdom and voices of many gay, lesbian, and transgender people, professionals, and activists I met in the course of my fieldwork. I do not pretend to represent their voices, but I hope my analysis helps uncover the workings of power—with its destructive and productive forces—in old age.

REFERENCES

Ramirez-Valles, J. Dirkes L., Berrett, H. (2014). *GayBy Boomers'* social support: exploring the connection between health and emotional and instrumental support in older gay men. *J. of Gerontological Social Work*, *57*, 218–234.

Rechy, J. (2013 [1963]). *City of night*. New York City, NY: Grove Press. [E-reader version].

Rowley, L. (2012, April 2). Baby Boomers will transform aging in america, panel says. *The Huffington Post*. Available: http://www.huffingtonpost.com/2012/04/02/aging-in-america-baby-boomers-arianna-huffington_n_1397686.html

ACKNOWLEDGMENTS

I am grateful to several LGBT organizations: Howard Brown Health Center; The Center on Halsted; Services & Advocacy for Gay, Lesbian, Bisexual, and Transgender Elders; the Chicago Task Force on LGBT Aging, and Prime Timers. They trusted me, opened their doors to me, and shared their expertise and resources with me.

I started thinking about *Queer Aging* during a fellowship I received at the Great Cities Institute of my home institution, the University of Illinois at Chicago. I completed the writing of this book during a Bellagio residency. I thank the Rockefeller Foundation for giving me, again, such a magnificent opportunity. *Muchas gracias de todo corazón* to Pilar Palacia, Managing Director, Bellagio Study and Conference Center. I feel extremely fortunate.

My gratitude extends to three research assistants who helped me during several stages of this project: Dianna Manjarrez, Jessica Dirkes, and Lucas Cardoso da Silva. Also,

Vanessa Fabbre and Chris Girman provided me critical feedback.

Last, I want to thank two amazing guys: my graciously aging husband, Brad Trask, and our son, Cameron. *Amor, gracias* for loving me, for cooking delicious meals, for arguing with me about my ideas (my husband and I do not always agree on queer politics), and for reading countless drafts. Cameron, thank you for helping me become a more loving human being. Watching you grow has enriched my appreciation for the aging marvel.

INTRODUCTION

When organizing the structure of *Queer Aging*, I aimed for simplicity. In the first chapter I review the existing research on older gay men and develop a framework for incorporating gerontology and queer theory (and its related sexuality studies). My point is to provide a critical perspective on the aging experience and the lenses through which we could better value the lives of older gay men. I then present the individual narratives of 11 gay men. They are not complete life histories, but accounts centered on the latter part of their life. In the closing chapter, I bring together the framework I outlined and these men's stories to continue queering gerontology.

QUEERING GERONTOLOGY

An Introduction

NOVEMBER 10, 2014: MY FRIEND ROBERT posted a selfie on Facebook and remarked, "*Tengo 55. . . . ¿Y ahora qué coño hago*?" [I'm 55. . . . What the heck do I do now?] The selfie shows his eyes looking down at the computer screen and his chin resting in his right hand—a pondering selfie. "Laugh at the world and be happy," a friend commented. Others followed: "Marry me." "But you don't look that age!" And "Sit by the window and wait for the end. . . . That's what I am doing, I am turning 47 in a couple of days . . . ." There is nothing extraordinary in Robert's meditative question and his friends' reactions. Yet, Robert's existential (and rhetorical) question conveys a transition, a beginning of a new phase—older age—and seeks a script to follow.

At the health club, my friend John asked, "Who is going to take care of me?" as he told me about his latest visit to his mother, who is in an assisted living facility in another city. John is also in his mid 50s, healthy and well-off. The fact that he is single worries him: "I might not find someone. I'm getting old and I'm single." John knows that in the gay world, the odds of finding a boyfriend or partner shrink considerably after the third decade of life. Although this is a valid concern, what has more weight for him is the possibility of not having the support and care he needs when his physical and mental abilities begin to dwindle. Our current healthcare and welfare system rests on the assumption that support comes from spouses, children, and siblings (usually women), and is unpaid. John is caring for his older mother and there is no one on the horizon to take care of him.

At the 2012 International AIDS conference, I witnessed a gay man speaking out angrily about his facial lipodystrophy to a panel of epidemiologists and physicians. He is 65 years old and runs a support group for older gay men living with HIV. He takes 14 pills throughout the morning and 11 at night. He makes the point that his health insurance covers almost all the treatment, all but the procedure to fix facial lipodystrophy: "A treatment that will stop me from looking like a skull."

In the meantime, four middle-age gay men try to defy aging in West Hollywood in the television show *Old Tricks and New Dogs*. The characters, poor replicas of those in *Sex & the City*—gay white males magically living a middle-class life—fight against the decay and paltriness of middle and old age by means that have become cliché: sex and lots of sex, penis obsession, Viagra, Botox, facelifts, pectoral augmentation, drugs, alcohol, and night clubs. In a revealing pool scene, even the youthful-looking Greg Louganis (a guest star in the show) executes a somersault dive.

These are some of the signs of a relatively new phenomenon: the older gay man. These are men of the Baby Boomer generation (whom I refer to as *Gayby Boomers*) who have reached what we call middle or old age, and who have aged with the self and collective "gay" identity like no other generation before (MetLife, 2010). The group is charting fairly novel territory. Like Robert, they are wondering what's next. Many of them are single, without close (physically and otherwise) relatives, childless, and aging along with their own "families of choice" (Bennett, 2008a). Yet, some of them are taking care of their parents and partners while preoccupied about where their own care will come from when their turn arrives (MetLife, 2010). Their appeal in our white gay male culture is also in decline as they face the unattractive space of older people. They are beginning to sketch out gay life after 50 (when we get our American Association for Retired Persons cards) in the same way their heterosexual Baby Boomer peers are redefining old age. The aging of this generation might be as world-shattering as the gay liberation and AIDS movements were (Heaphy, 2007; Weinstein, 2007).

As they have been for the past 40 years, older gay men are trapped between expressing who they are and the stigma toward gender nonconformity, HIV and AIDS, and old age. Homophobia remains a real threat: "We're going to be living with the same bigots who hated as when we were younger"—an older lesbian warned us about assisted living facilities in a meeting of senior lesbian, gay, bisexual, and transgender (LGBT) people. Yet, they are creating structures and paths to define life as an older gay person. One participant in this book project told me, "My generation probably lost a lot of people, but the ones of us that are left are sort of defining what it means to be older because we are out. We are trying to figure out what it means to be an older gay man." These men are relying on existing cultural scripts and social structures, as well as the habits they gathered throughout the course of their lives as Gayby Boomers. In *Queer Aging*, I propose that Gayby Boomers are challenging stereotypes about older gay people, shifting the meanings of old age, exposing and questioning some of the heterosexual foundations of old age, and, simultaneously, reproducing other features of heterosexual and racial systems embedded in our neoliberal capitalist world.

Queer Aging features stories of older gay men of the Baby Boomer generation and the ways in which they are changing old age and gerontology (the study of old age). The stories I have curated methodologically come from single, partnered, and divorced men; black, Latino, and white men; men who are living with HIV and men who are not; and men who are primary caregivers for others. The narratives address how older gay men navigate the cultural discourses and social norms about aging and being gay to construct their own lives—their sense of self, social spaces, and health. They also speak to the shortcomings of the dominant (heteronormative) gerontology field, our understanding of old age and the policies and services derived from it, and the possibilities of change—what I call *queer gerontology*. I argue, based on the voices of these men, that although the recent visibility of the older gay male subject is an important step against discrimination, it also reinforces (heterosexual) norms about aging and masculinity that might, unintentionally, subjugate gay men and actually create undue stress on them. I dispute the call for "rights" and inclusion of older LGBT people and propose we pause and reflect critically on the identities we are promoting and their consequences.

THE EMERGENCE OF THE GAYBY BOOMERS

The overall population in Western societies is aging at a faster rate than ever before (World Health Organization, 2014). In the United States, the older gay male population is growing rapidly, mainly as a result of the aging of the Baby Boomer generation—those born between 1946 and 1964 (Pew Research Center, 2014). Within Baby Boomers, there is a group of gay men—Gayby Boomers—who are different from their heterosexual Boomers and the larger gay male population (Funders for Lesbian and Gay Issues, 2004; Grossman, 2008; Herdt & de Vries, 2004). This is the first group of men to embrace the "gay" identity. This cohort was involved actively in the gay liberation movement. Many in this group began to live openly with their partners or significant others and create large communities, particularly in major U.S. urban centers (D'Emilio, 1998). Then, the AIDS epidemic erupted during the early 1980s, setting back the collective gains of the gay liberation movement and changing its agenda (Crimp, 2002). Actually, AIDS postponed aging for many gay men. If old age was already hidden in the gay male culture, the thought of getting older was suspended. In the midst of the mounting number of deaths and infections, this generation mobilized, again, to fight the epidemic. Now, with the help of antiretroviral therapies (ARTs), imagining old age resumed and many Gayby Boomers are the first to age with HIV (Bennett, 2008a). In 2011, about one quarter of the people living with HIV in the United States was 55 years and older (Center for Disease Control and Prevention, 2015). The life expectancy (and its quality) of those gay men living with HIV/AIDS has expanded and now they are becoming part of the general aging population. Thus, Gayby Boomers have taken a unique path. Their milestones and life transitions are different from those of the majority—dating, college, job, marriage, parenthood and grandparenthood, divorce, caregiving, and retirement.

The contemporary appearance of the older gay male subject and population, in the larger society as well as within gay communities, is not only numerical, but also social and cultural. A discourse around older LGBT people has emerged in the United States within the past decade. Communities and grassroots organizations of older gay (or homosexual) men have existed for much longer than that, of course. For most of the 20th century we lived with the stereotypical image of old gay men as loners who were depressed and sexual perverts (Kimmel, Rose, Orel, & Greene, 2006). Today's visibility is different—a "positive" and respectable older gay male subject, a post-AIDS or by-product of the AIDS epidemic.

The leading organization in setting the contemporary agenda of the older LGBT population is Services and Advocacy for Gay, Lesbian, Bisexual, and Transgender Elders (SAGE), which was founded in 1978 by a small group in New York City. Its initial name was Senior Action in a Gay Environment and the primary drive was creating social and educational activities. The first group is featured in *Silent Pioneers* (Marks & Winer, 1985), a 1980s documentary aimed at challenging the negative stereotypes of older gays and lesbians.

Small professional associations around LGBT people and gerontology started to appear during the late 1970s (Kimmel et al., 2006). One example is the National Association for Lesbian and Gay Gerontology, which held the first national Conference on Gay and Lesbian Aging in

1981(Keppel & Firestein, 2007). The Lesbian and Gay Aging Issues Network emerged around the same time within the American Society on Aging (Kimmel et al., 2006). It was recognized formally by the American Society on Aging in 1994 (Keppel & Firestein, 2007), and its name later extended to LGBT Aging Issues Network. These groups raised questions about the inclusion of sexual orientation and the importance of sexuality within fairly conservative circles of researchers and professionals in gerontology. Their efforts led to an official recommendation to include LGBT people under the umbrella category of "minority populations" in the 2005 White House Conference on Aging (Knauer, 2011). The American Association for Retired Persons then began partnering with LGBT organizations, included LGBT persons in its diversity and inclusion policies, and now it provides a range of resources to LGBT seniors—from financial to leisure to dating (Knauer, 2011).

A strong impetus for the formation and spread of a discourse on older gay men came from the Obama administration's inclusion of LGBT in health and social services for aging. In 2010, the Department of Health and Human Services funded the first national resource center for older LGBT persons. The purpose of this center is to provide information, training, and services to support the health of LGBT people who are 60 years of age and older. The center is led by SAGE, which created a network of 23 affiliates in 16 states to deliver services to older LGBT people (SAGE, n.d. a). As mentioned, SAGE provides a variety of services: social support groups, classes, unemployment and financial assistance, and housing. Initiave was followed by a 2011 report from the Institute of Medicine calling for research on older gay men's health (Institute of Medicine of the National

Academies, 2011). What is more, in 2015, the American Geriatrics Society put forward a position statement demanding equal treatment of older LGBT people in medical settings, assisted living facilities, and health research (American Geriatrics Society Ethics Committee, 2015).

Significantly, this push for attention for older LGBT people coincided with the marriage equality movement, supporting each other. The *New York Times*, for example, ran a story of two men (ages 77 years and 86 years) being married while in the hospital after 39 years of being together (Hartocollis, 2011). This image of an older (read, "de-sexed") gay couple getting married certainly appeals to our popular notions of love and justice.

Around the same time, we began to see images and stories about older gay men in the popular media. In 2007, the *New York Times* published a story titled, "Aging and Gay, and Facing Prejudice in Twilight" (Gross, 2007). And the following year, Newsweek (Bennett, 2008b) added two related stories on the invisibility of LGBT elders and the aging of HIV patients. This time, the stories showed gay men (and lesbians) as the victims of stigma toward sexual minorities and older people. The loneliness, poor health, and financial troubles they encounter are not of their own making, but the outcome of social exclusion. Also, in 2010, the film *Beginners* (Urdang et al., and Mills, 2010) portrayed an older man coming out as gay after the death of his wife. The film won an Oscar and was actually well-liked by mainstream audiences. And in 2014, PBS began broadcasting the British sitcom *Vicious*, which centers on an elderly gay couple who has been together for almost 50 years.

All these new stories, from popular media to government mandates and nonprofit organizations, seek the inclusion of the senior LGBT person into mainstream society. There are few exceptions, for sure. In the 2011 movie *The Best Exotic Marigold Hotel* (*for the Elderly & Beautiful*, as the full title reads), for example, the gay male character, a retired British judge, suddenly dies after meeting again the Indian man he loved in his youth. His former lover is married to a woman—a path he was supposedly forced to take after the male young lovers were discovered. The death of the gay character here underscores the exclusion from the "elderly and beautiful"; it reminds us of the tragic consequences of same-sex desire.

This visibility and actual physical presence of the older gay male figure raises a variety of questions: How does one live as an older gay person? How do the subjective views of older gay men relate to the images in popular media, government policies, and scientific gerontological literature? Do those images reflect the (potential) diversity of the experiences of these men? How do gay men deal with the societal expectations around old age, such as "successful aging," homophobia, and the stigma of old age? And what kinds of unique circumstances does the intersection of race, social class, and HIV status create in old age?

The entrance of the current cohort of older gay men into the aging population, and the questions I just raised, are relevant because of the strikingly heterosexual (and asexual) configuration of gerontology (Brown, 2009). Gerontology does not know about queer aging (National Gay and Lesbian Task Force, 2005; Thompson, 1994). The literature in this field (as I address later in this chapter) is rooted in a variety of assumptions about self, desire, coupling, family, masculinity, community, and life course emerging mostly from a heterosexual, white, middle-class world. Again, this is about to change simply because older LGBT people are forcing the field to adjust by their sheer manifestation in numbers and, even more, by their activism.

A quick look at the LGBT and queer academic body of literature raises an analogous difficulty. Scholars of LGBT studies have largely overlooked the uniqueness of old age (with few exceptions [e.g., Heaphy, 2007]). Although encouraging a critical analysis of heterosexuality, they have not yet dealt with age as a status and phenomenon. Age is one of the axes of social organization, together with race, gender, and social class (Plummer, 2010); and age is not only a biological process, but also a social and cultural one (Twigg, 2004). Likewise, scholars have usually combined all age groups (for an exception, see Fredriksen-Goldsen, Kim, Shiu, Goldsen, and Emlet [2015]), ignoring what life course perspective and gerontology have argued: that cohort, history, and context matter in the experience of aging. We must not assume, following this contention, that the experience of old age is uniform among gay men (or men who express same-sex desire). Social class position, racial location, cohort, and HIV produce variations.

In *Queer Aging*, my ultimate goal is to contribute to the transformation of conventional gerontology and sexuality/queer studies through the examination of the subjective experiences of a group of Gayby Boomers. In an iterative process, I look at the stories of these men through the lenses of sexuality, queer theory, and aging (including the life course approach) while using the insights I gain to adjust these same lenses. I propose that we need to put these multiple perspectives in dialogue to exchange, revise, and develop conceptual tools that could assist us in analyzing and changing the new realities of old age.

As I analyze the lives of Gayby Boomers, I am also aware that subject and social practices are not constituted solely by sexuality or ideas about sexual desire. As Kayal (1994) warns us: "It is inappropriate to see people primarily in terms of their sexual activity" (p. 411). Sexual activity and sexual orientation may be relevant only when they become political issues—hence, forces shaping peoples' lives. There are discourses and habits about race and social class that come into play. In *Queer Aging*, I incorporate the voices of men who identify as black, Latino, and white from different social positions and, within these groups, I highlight the stories of those living with HIV/AIDS. I am looking for the ways in which sexuality in old age might intersect with race and social class.

I am equally mindful of the intricacies involved by my reliance on the concepts of "Baby Boomer" and "queer." The scholarly and popular use of Baby Boomers frequently refers to (unquestioned) cultural elements (and even marketing strategies), ignoring the roles of race and social class (Katz & Marshal, 2003). The risk is to assign primacy to cultural and discursive practices. Part of my project, as noted earlier, is to bring the materiality of race and social class into the analysis of Gayby Boomers' lives. Regarding the term *queer*, I rely on the definition by Warner (1999): it refers to the multiple ways in which "people can find themselves at odds" with white heterosexual culture (p. 38). This notion is at the heart of queer theory and encourages us to look beyond identities (e.g., gay man). It does not deny the value of identities, but emphasizes the relations of power embedded in the lives of Gayby Boomers. (I elaborate on this point in subsequent sections.) I also mean it to be inclusive of the various sexualities among the male participants in this study. Most of them call themselves gay, but a close reading of their stories (as is seen in later chapters) reveals nuances and divergences. Therefore, when I write "gay," it is for practical purposes only.

Although my project emerges from very particular social and cultural settings—the United States—it has further implications. The call to assert the "human rights" of the LGBT person is now on the agenda of nations around the globe—rich and poor—and international agencies such as the United Nations and World Health Organization. This agenda has been defined largely by groups from Western (and predominantly white) societies; hence, it contains notions about same-sex desire specific to such sites. Some scholars and activists from non-Western and poor societies reject this dominant LGBT rights agenda because it silences the diversity of practices and identities of men outside the West (Massad, 2002). It has the danger (if not its purpose) of colonizing local cultures. It is plausible the increased visibility of older LGBT persons in the West, and the subsequent incorporation of "older" into the LGBT rights agenda, will take a similar path, as LGBT organizations recognize the vulnerability of their older cohorts. It is imperative, therefore, to examine critically notions of older gay men—or men who love or desire men—that are emerging in the West as they might propagate beyond that.

In what follows, I offer a framework, queer gerontology, to describe and analyze the lived experiences of older Gayby Boomers. I first present and probe the prevailing gerontological research, which unavoidably takes us to issues of health and "successful aging." I then build a critique of the predominant gerontological research on older gay men and develop an outline for queer gerontology. I conclude this introductory chapter with a methodological note explaining my use of gay men's life stories as the primary data source.

SUCCESSFUL AGING: GERONTOLOGY'S VIEWS ON GAY MEN

During the past 25 years, only about 28 scientific articles have been published exclusively on older gay and lesbian populations (Fredriksen-Goldsen & Muraco, 2010). The story emerging from this narrow body of literature follows the same plot of the larger LGBT movement outlined by John D'Emilio (2014). It's a narrative about heroism: confronting oppression, creating community, and gaining recognition. It underscores a move from older gay men being silenced (at best) and thought of as depressed and lonely people to an image of men striving to age successfully, defying the prevalent societal stigma. The early literature, during the 1970s and part of the 1980s (e.g., Berger, 1982; Cruz, 2003; Kelly, 1977; Kimmel et al., 2006), responded primarily to then-widespread homophobic discourse (Hughes, 2006). It had major limitations because it relied mostly on quantitative data (with very few exceptions), and on convenient and small samples of mainly white, relatively well-off, and socially connected men. Scholars then put forward a different picture: a positive gay identity; older gay people do create "families of choice" and communities, and their struggles in old age are largely a result of societal forces not of their own homosexual making (De Vries & Hoctel, 2006; Herdt, Beeler, & Rwals, 1997; McMahon, 2003). The most recent research is framed by the concepts of successful aging and health disparities (e.g., Fredriksen-Goldsen et al., 2015; Friend, 1990; Krehely, 2009). Ironically, it continues to present the aging experience of gay men as a pathology (as my summary of such research shows next).

Mainstream gerontological research tells us that older gay men face unique and critical negative health outcomes that prevent them from aging successfully, including limited social connections, poor mental health, risk for HIV infection, and substance use. Social support, we are told, is crucial in older age (White, Philogene, Fine & Sinha, 2009). For gay men (even those living with HIV), for example, social support may buffer stigmatization and enhance wellbeing (D'Augelli, Grossman, Hershberger, & O'Connell, 2001; de Vries & Hoctel, 2004; Chesney, Chambers, Taylor, & Johnson, 2003). Older gay men, however, have limited social support and are twice as likely as their heterosexual peers to live alone (Bennett, 2008a; Fredriksen-Goldsen et al., 2013; Grossman, D'Augelli, & Hershberger, 2000; Shippy, Cantor, & Brennan, 2004). Among white older gay men, friends are the most common source of support, followed by partners and biological families, unlike the rest of the population in which biological family is the most common source of support (Herdt et al., 1997; Lyons, Pitts, Grierson, Thorpe & Power, 2010; Metlife, Lesbian and Gay Aging Issues Network of the American Society of Aging, & Zogby International, 2006; Shippy et al., 2004; White et al., 2009).

Gay men, it is said, are at elevated risk for mental health disorders, such as depression, and substance and alcohol abuse (Fredriksen-Goldsen et al., 2013; Lewis, 2009; Wallace, Cochran, Durazo & Ford, 2011). In selective samples, up to one third of older gay men report depressive symptoms—more than double the rate in the general older male population, and the percent could be higher among those with HIV (Raws, 2004; Shippy et al., 2004; Steffens, Fisher, Langa,

Potter, & Plassman, 2009; Vance, McGuinness, Musgrove, Orel, & Fazeli, 2011). In the limited data available, it is estimated that 11% have a drinking problem and 17% have other substance use problems (D'Augelli et al., 2001; Grossman et al., 2000).

Epidemiological studies tell us that older gay men, regardless of HIV status, continue an active sexual life (Jimenez, 2003; Lovejoy et al., 2008; Raws, 2004). They, too, alert us that the HIV prevalence in the group can be as high as 14% (Dolcini, Catania, Stall, & Pollack, 2003; Jimenez, 2003; Lovejoy et al., 2008; Raws, 2004). Of course, the risk for HIV infection reduces with age. HIV, notably, is thought to accelerate the "physiological" aging process of gay men. It triggers psychological distress and a decrease in social support, which may aggravate illnesses common in old age (Chesney et al., 2003; Cooperman, Arnsten, & Klein, 2007; Heckman et al., 2000; Raws, 2004; Vance et al., 2011). HIV can also increase frailty, functional performance, arthritis, cardiovascular diseases, and kidney and liver diseases (Casau, 2005; Effros et al., 2008; High et al., 2012).

From a psychosocial perspective, researchers maintain that stigma toward homosexuality, people living with HIV, and older age poses undue stress on older gay men (D'Augelli & Grossman, 2001; Kertzner, 2001; McMahon, 2003). Older gay men, for instance, report pervasive homophobia in health and social services, and age discrimination in gay communities (de Vries & Hoctel, 2006; Gray & Dressel, 1985; Jackson, Johnson, & Roberts, 2008; Johnson, Jackson, Arnette, & Koffman, 2005; Kertzner, 2001), while those living with HIV still fear disclosing their status (Emlet, 2007, 2008; Vance et al., 2011).

ACCELERATED AGING VERSUS CRISIS COMPETENCY

Given the unique life course of gay men and their marginalization, gerontologists have put forward two possible aging scenarios: accelerated aging versus crisis competency (or mastery aging). The first one suggests the markers of aging (e.g., functional and health decline) appear earlier in gay men than in their counterparts because of a life span of stigmatization (de Vries & Blando, 2004). This also may be the particular case of gay men living with HIV, whose aging might be both accelerated and exacerbated because of the virus, the medical therapies, and their combined side effects (Casau, 2005; Effros et al., 2008; France, 2009).

The counterview, crisis competency, indicates gay men are actually better equipped to face aging because of the skills they have acquired through confronting marginalization—and the AIDS epidemic (e.g., Berger, 1982; Cruz, 2003; David & Knight, 2008; Quam & Whitford, 1992; Wight, LeBlanc, de Vries & Detels, 2012). Their age clock might also extend their youth or adulthood, and even blur those age distinctions because they do not live the normative milestones such as marriage and parenthood (Bennett, 2008b).

Whether gay men are at a disadvantage or advantage compared with heterosexual males is difficult to ascertain, and beyond my purpose here. What I want to point out is that this perspective, which is centered squarely in gerontology, sees both aging and sexual difference as pathologies—still. Beneath it all is an assumption that both health and medical conditions can be modified to avoid illness and disease, and to achieve "healthy aging," which takes us to the dominant theme in contemporary gerontology: successful aging.

SUCCESSFUL AGING

The agenda of successful aging was first introduced by Rowe and Kahn in their 1987 article in the journal *Science*. They propose that the effects of aging (e.g., weakened functionality, depression, heart disease) are not natural or fully attributed to age, but are also caused by lifestyle and environmental elements, such as diet, exercise, social support, and living conditions. We must, they suggest, distinguish between "normal" or usual and *successful* aging. The former being those consequences intrinsic to age and the latter being the ability to extend physical and mental functioning until the point of death. The assertion is that the aches—bodily, intellectual, and financial—we experience with age are (basically) of our own making and that, with this sense of personal responsibility, comes also the possibility of freeing oneself from such degeneration. Note that, although they claim a factual or medical distinction between intrinsic and acquired aging, they unknowingly endorse the idea that old age is constructed socially. If we follow their logic, the division is faulty. What is thought of as natural today (e.g., memory loss) will become acquired after the next medical, dietary, or technological discovery.

Rowe and Khan (1987) identify two factors as crucial to successful aging: autonomy and social support. The first one refers to a sense of control and independence. Arguably, they allow us to control our destiny, hence to deter illness and disease. We must strive to be self-sufficient. Social support, the second factor, increases the ability to fight disease and decay by providing companionship, assistance, and even financial means. Social support, however, must not lessen autonomy. We should not "do for" others, but rather facilitate and encourage autonomy and individual control. Gerontologists have since then expanded this basic idea. They argue that older people must engage in "productive" activities (e.g., volunteering, exercising) to sustain health (Muscik & Wilson, 2008; Willigen, 2000). Strictly speaking, from a health and medicine stance, they now pinpoint three core components of successful aging: minimizing risk for disease and disability via self-management, maintaining physical and intellectual functions, and sustaining social support and civic engagement (Andersen & Prohaska, 2014).

Successful aging awakened an interest in sex; older people are not seen as lacking sexual desire anymore (Hinchliff, 2009). Toward the end of the 20th century, sexual activity in older age started to be encouraged as crucial for healthy aging. In our consumer economy and popular culture, successful aging has then come to indicate strong, active bodies; full, white smiles; sexual prowess; encore careers; travel; and financial independence (Calasanti & King, 2005). With this doctrine, Baby Boomers have championed the idea that aging can be resisted and deferred, and that people can control their bodies and lives through consumption and lifestyle choices (Higgs & McGowan, 2012).

Gerontologists working on LGBT populations soon embraced this concept without questioning it. In his 1991 pioneering paper, Friend (1990) recommends "positive" identity as the basis for LGBT people's successful aging. By *positive* he means a self and collective "affirming" identity as a gay male, free of any homophobic residues. He maintains that men who remain in the closet or manage their identity otherwise have difficulty adjusting to old age, whereas those who have accomplished an affirmative identity have acquired "crisis competency." The notion of aging successfully is also now championed in the HIV field (High et al., 2012; Kahana & Kahana, 2001; Vance et al., 2011).

SAGE has made successful aging a core of its mission: "We believe that all LGBT people deserve to age financially secure, free from discrimination and surrounded by the people they love and the supports they need. With proper planning and a new frame of mind, aging can engender new possibilities and the realization of long-held dreams" (SAGE, n.d. b). Following this stance, SAGE (2014) recently conducted a market research survey among older LGBT people. The main findings, not surprisingly, include concerns about homophobia, financial security, lack of physical attractiveness, and loneliness, along with a desire to travel, volunteer, join social groups, and work on hobbies. Indeed, many gay men in their 50s and older base their self-worth on sex, physical attraction, conquering younger men, body image, and financial security (Hajek, 2014).

Although I do not discount the core research and practice of gerontology, and although I actually advocate for older (and young) people's ability to live a full life, I contest this prevailing paradigm. My account is different, as are the stories that men shared with me. Their experiences of aging are not confined to illness, disease, and stigmatization, and to a utilitarian pursuit of health until death—or successful aging.

The body of knowledge I outlined here lacks a sociocultural context and queer perspectives, focused narrowly on illness (or its absence) and function (Estes, 2001). Even within the canons of empirical health research, the available "evidence" is constrained in scope. The samples are small and comprised mostly of white males, age cohorts are not differentiated, and the gay identity is rarely defined or just limited to a self-identification. It is not only that the identity "gay man" goes unexamined, but that in doing so it is reaffirmed as an unproblematic, monolithic, and universal category. Such a view underscores the dichotomy of gay–heterosexual, either overtly when making empirical comparisons among groups (e.g., Fredriksen-Goldsen et al., 2013) or indirectly when focusing solely on gay people as a uniform group (I take on the fluidity and porosity of sex and gender identities in the following section). More significant, the weight of successful aging creates an unrealistic social expectation to be "healthy" and "independent" on older folks and reiterates individual responsibility (over collective) in the quest for well-being.

In *Queer Aging* I rely on men's subjective experiences to understand how sexuality, race, and age work. The story I tell is about the taken-for-granted and almost invisible forces of power embedded in the gay identity and the lives of gay men in old age. How is "gay" defined? What is the meaning of old age? How do race and sexuality intersect? How does the subjective view resemble (or not) the broader gerontological discourse of successful aging? What are the consequences of visibility? Those are the questions I am interested in addressing because they are not being asked and because their answers will help us inform mainstream heteronormative gerontology.

QUEER GERONTOLOGY

Queer gerontology is a critical analysis of the heterosexual norms shaping scholarship and practice in gerontology. This approach is relatively new, with only a handful of authors writing about it (Hughes, 2006), and so it remains fairly unexplored. Queer gerontology is a strategy, more than a concept, to raise questions, develop methodologies, gather data, and create new theoretical tools. It works as a set of lenses to look at aging. The goal is to unmask the ways in which heterosexual dominant norms define what it means to be an older person—from the decline of our bodies to retirement, support communities, and living conditions. It implies making visible same-sex desire, love, and relationships in old age, and documenting the manner in which older queer people live. The interest of queer gerontology is not limited to heterosexuality (or sexuality); it comprises racial and political systems to the extent that they are connected with heterosexuality reinforcing one another (Ferguson, 2004; Heaphy, 2007).

I pose queer gerontology as a framework to read the narratives of Gayby Boomers. As I began listening to their stories, I realized the constraints of traditional gerontology and the need to bring insights from the scholarship on queer studies and critical gerontology to start making sense of them. The lives these men have constructed do not follow the traditional path. Their experiences in older age are not limited to illness and disease; their marginalization is not new and not only attributed to old age. Rather, their lives are about being in the margins (sometimes feeling content there and others times not) and about the forces of heterosexuality, race, capitalism, gay liberation, and AIDS. They are not about achieving successful aging, but about coping with the unrealistic demands and limits such a goal imposes on them to live a full life.

In the words of John D'Emilio (2014), queer theory is a turn—from focusing our inquiry on sexual minorities or LGBT experience to analyzing the center: heterosexuality.

We must leave our "ghetto," he asks us, and insert queerness into heterosexual history and social structures. "If we embed queer stories in a larger political economy, a larger national political history, they will become less separated and less self-ghettoized, and instead become seen as integral to, more connected to, and more essential for understanding broader narratives of US history" (p. 228). Although previous LGBT history and sociology works were based on an idea of "liberation" of LGBT people, the emphasis of queer scholars' examination is on heterosexuality and on how its own rationality produces marginal spaces and identities, such as homosexuality and bisexuality (Green, 2007).

Queer theory means to investigate the manner in which discursive practices create identities and how, or if, heteronormativity shapes our daily lives and social institutions (Gamson & Moon, 2004; Green, 2007). Yet, heterosexuality is not assumed to be unadulterated, but porous and unstable. Our sexual categories are not natural, but are created socially (Valocchi, 2005), and the binary sets of, say, male–female, gay–heterosexual, young–old are not dichotomies, but only spaces by which lived experience is constrained (Stein & Plummer, 1994).

The distrust of LGBT identities emerged from Foucault (1995; Green, 2007). He argued against the idea of an "essential" human nature, proposing that the social phenomena we study—gay and aging, for example—are fully constituted by discourses such as psychiatry and medicine. These discourses (or "sciences," academic disciplines) provide a framework to understand the inner and external parts of the object of interest. They do not hide a true meaning, but create meaning. The homosexual subject, consequently, is the product of a fairly recent discourse around sexuality, in which homosexuality was created in opposition to heterosexuality. This new prominence of homosexuality in scientific and medical fields served only to assert heterosexuality. The gay identity, later developed in the United States (Chauncey, 1994), was born out of this discursive separation of sexual desire. It became the only signifier of same-sex male desire. In our everyday life, gay grew into a uniting identity for thousands of men, while being suffocating and reductionist at the same time. Gay, contrary to common belief, is not subversive in and of itself, but rather is a part of the networks of power that manage sexual desire.

The visibility of gayness, by underscoring difference and diversity, reinforces and naturalizes the homo–hetero, male–female distinction and heightens the superiority of the heterosexual male position. It also erodes same-sex desires that do not fit into such "sexual epistemology" (Massad, 2002, p. 363). My argument in this book, therefore, is not about bringing to light the "invisible" and "repressed" stories of old gay men. What I claim is that the aging experience of these men cannot be fully understood as "gay," and that it actually challenges our notions of gayness, exposing its racial and social class basis. The contemporary visibility of older LGBT subject, moreover, needs to be problematized.

If we think of our gender and sexual identities as being socially constructed, then our work as scholars and practitioners in gerontology is not about advocating for "rights" but about inspecting how and which identities are being fashioned and advanced, and with what consequences (Hughes, 2006; Warner, 1999). The call for rights implies an effort and a desire to assimilate in a analogous way that the positioning of gay as a "minority" reinstates heterosexuality as the guiding code (Stein & Plummer, 1994).

Following postmodernism, queer theory also questions rationality as a practice of power (Stein & Plummer, 1994). Heterosexuality is based on a time defined by biological reproduction and its assigned consequences: marriage and family. Of course, there are fractures (Binnie & Klesse, 2012) within such normative time, especially as we see the number of single mothers and childless couples grow, and as marriage is delayed. From this biological phenomenon, a rationality about work and progress has been created to organize our lives under capitalism in the West. Our bodies and time must not be idle; they need to be disciplined, productive, and efficient. The queer stand, then, invites us to suspend our belief on the naturalness of coupledom, marriage, family, work, progress, and historical time as they are intertwined with heterosexuality (Castiglia & Reed, 2011; Freeman, 2010; Halberstam, 2005).

Taking the position to its fullest, queer theory rejects the existence of the subject (e.g., older gay male). It pursues "subjectless" politics (Green, 2007). Likewise, it skips the material reality and the social nature of life and identities. I believe this is dangerous because it denies the possibility of an actor—a subject making decisions. I rather rely on the insights from Foucault (1995) and two strands of sociology: constructivism and symbolic interactionism. The subject (e.g., old person, gay male) does not exist naturally, or a priori, but it is created through discourses (e.g., medicine, psychiatry) and social interaction (Green, 2007; Valocchi, 2005). The bounds and potentials of such a given subject are defined through these same discourses and interactions.

In *Aberrations in Black*, Roderick Ferguson (2004) gives us a foundation for a queer of color analysis—or to bring race and queer relations together. In the same manner, we discard a monolithic identity of gay, we must do so for race: "Queer of color critique employs cultural forms to bear witness to the critical gender and sexual heterogeneity that comprises minority cultures" (p. 24). There is no "black" or "Latino" nature. A sense of blackness, for example, does not come from skin color; rather, it gets attached to it. Our current racial configuration, Ferguson and others argued (Roediger, 1991), is the outcome of the formation of the state and its capitalist economy in the United States. This origin makes it difficult to disentangle sexuality, race, and gender. We cannot fully appreciate the aging of older men without an analysis of gender, race, and social class. As an exercise on the social construction of race, I invite you to "find race" in the *Queer Aging* narratives. The race of each man, most likely, will materialize in socioeconomic circumstances, family structure, history with education and religious institutions, and even in his encounter with AIDS.

A Queer View on Successful Aging

Our contemporary images of old age are dominated by a fear of aging, and this does not exclude gay men. In our white, middle-class context, aging and dying are dreaded. Intellectuals and journalists speak of such anxieties (Kreider, 2013; Slevin, 2008). We isolate the old (as we do with the ill); parents and grandparents do not live among us, the young. The old is an unattractive and unproductive body: weak, ill, a failure. In promoting this view, youth and health take prominence as eternal states of being. The act of dying itself has being removed further from us to hospitals and health-care professionals.

Concomitant to such notion of old age, and perhaps because of that, we have the successful aging manifesto (Sandberg, 2008). These two impulses are actually complementary: only if we think of old age as decay and a problem can we consider "positive" aging. In both instances, as I alluded to already, the self as a moral and responsible subject are at play, and both are grounded on a normative view of the body and time—productive and efficient (Castiglia & Reed, 2011). Moreover, the seemingly conflicting views are informed by medicine and our consumer culture, which continues to dominate gerontology (Katz & Marshal, 2003; Powell & Biggs, 2003).

Successful aging also emphasizes independency, strength, and continuation (rather than decline or rupture [Fabbre, 2015; Powell & Biggs, 2003]). And it offers solutions to the dwindling body: diet and exercise, volunteering and encore careers, sex and drugs to enhance sexual activity (focused on the penis and penetration), and face and body surgical lifts. Older men—gay and otherwise—have internalized these notions (Slevin, 2008). We are encouraged to take on this regime to feel better (read, young) about ourselves at any cost. We are expected to engage actively in practices to delay the appearance of the signs of aging (Higgs & McGowan, 2012). Body enhancement products and surgeries once the domain of women are now targeted to and consumed by men (Leonard, Duncan, & Barrett, 2012).

At the cultural and individual levels, successful aging has become a hegemonic idea and a disciplinary activity (Calasanti & King, 2005; Estes, 2001; Slevin, 2008). It is not that it rejects an older way of aging—a "natural" way of aging; it creates a new "natural" way of being old, a new ethics of old age. With this comes a moral imperative: "not to let one's self go" (Higgs & McGowan, 2012, p. 26). Those who fail, who "let themselves go," are weak and lack individual responsibility (Katz & Marshal, 2003; Slevin, 2008). This new moral also relieves others, including the state, from people's care and well-being—as it was the case with AIDS during the 1980s and 1990s. We brought illness and financial insecurity upon ourselves; hence, we are undeserving of care (Powell, 2004).

Thus, today, older people can create a sense of themselves by means of good health (e.g., diet, exercise), counseling (e.g., therapy and support groups), physical alterations (Powell, 2004), and finances (e.g., independency, retirement)—as in the successful aging creed. These are what Foucault referred to as "technologies of the self" (Foucault, 1998; Powell, 2004). They are the means by which we both think of and present ourselves to the outside world. In them lie the constraints and possibilities for the self.

For gay men, the attention to sexuality brought by successful aging might be welcome. Yet, this new emphasis is added to an already existing preoccupation with youth, sex, and consumerism in gay culture (Leonard et al., 2013). It pressures, even more, gay men to align with this sexuality in older age discourse, hence to use biomedicine and other tools to stay sexually attractive and active. It pushes them to buy goods and services to remain young, fit, and virile (Leonard et al., 2013; Slevin, Thomas & Linneman, 2010).

The conversations I had with gay men reflect ambivalence about successful aging. Men experience a sense of freedom to enjoy a sexual life in older age. They talk about sex, pursue sexual partners, and benefit from the drugs for erectile dysfunction. Some of them do feel better about themselves when they exercise. In contrast, men judge themselves and others negatively for the way they look: their bodies, face, and hair. Some of them try to "improve" their looks through beauty products and surgeries. They blame themselves (and others) for not being financially secure. Other gay men, including those living with HIV, struggle to achieve physical health and are overwhelmed by everyday financial and family demands. Some reject the messages about safe sex. Many regret being single; they think of themselves as failing to build an intimate, long-lasting relationship. A few men do not think of themselves as gay or queer; they do not base their self-concept in sexual orientation terms. And last, I heard how men feel left out; their collective memories and history are ignored by young gay men, and certainly the larger society.

The Social Construction of Aging

Beyond the contemporary idea of aging successfully, how we think of and experience aging is shaped by two primary forces: medicine and capitalism (Wallach & Brotman, 2013). There are other institutions and structures implicated in the construction of old age: work, schooling, welfare, healthcare, marriage, and gender. Yet, since the early 20th century, medicine took over, and then our capitalist mode of production followed. For instance, Estes (2001) notes that the devaluation of aging is largely caused by the separation between home and workplace, retirement, and replacement of senior employees with younger, less costly, ones (see also Laws [1993]).

Aging as a "problem" that needed to be studied and fixed by medicine emerged during the 1930s (Estes & Binney, 1989). Sex is a conspicuous instance. During the early and mid 20th century, lack of sexual activity and desire were part of normal age decay. Then, it became sexual dysfunction for which technologies were developed and sold so that men could continue performing sexually (Katz and Marshal, 2003). Parenthetically, masculinity, the penis, and sex were reinforced and lengthened to our later years. Older age became medicalized. Although medicine has extended life expectancy and (sometimes) quality of life, it has placed control and power in the hands of "experts" and a market economy (Powell, 2004). Medicalization implies treating the experience as a pathology or an illness, and designing policies and programs based on such assumptions (Estes, 2001; Estes & Binney, 1989). Given the medical model, one outcome is the understanding of old age as the "problem" of the individual (Estes, 2001). Another result is the creation of a whole consumer market for cosmetic surgery and biomedical products to manage the body, the wrinkled skin, and male virility (Higgs & McGowan, 2012). Scholars refer to this as the "aging enterprise" and the "commodification of aging" (Estes, 2001). The former describes an industry for the production, selling, and consumption of the aging experience. It includes physicians and psychologists; medical, pharmaceutical, and leisure businesses; and, of course, us, the consumers (Katz, 2000; Katz & Marshal, 2003). The latter, commodity, is the outcome of the former. Aging is a product exchanged in the marketplace.

The commodification of aging is highlighted in gay men's lives because of the centrality of sex. Gay seniors are desexualized in a hypersexualized culture (Knauer, 2011), and this is especially visible in "gay spaces" (Green, 2008)—the venues and neighborhoods gay men have secured for their own safety. Yet, acquiring and sustaining these spaces has been based on consumption, sex, and physical attractiveness (Heaphy, 2007; Jones & Pugh, 2005). Even more, in gay spaces there are hierarchies of attractiveness influencing access to sexual partners and social support. Older gay men are then compelled to participate in the aging enterprise (Ellies, 2009). In what seems to work as a self-sustaining system, the centrality of sex (especially the penis), the body, and masculinity are then perpetuated.

The Aging Body

The corporeal quality of our lives is at the core of aging. The body is where discourses and practices about aging are reinforced or contested—and intersected with those of social class, gender, and race (Cronin & King, 2010; Slevin, 2008; Wallach & Brotman, 2013). In the post-AIDS era, the idealized gay male body is a display of masculinity: lean, muscular, athletic, and clean-cut (at least in theory) through physical exercise (Drummond, 2006; Jones & Pugh 2005). This is only a slight variation from the body propagated before AIDS: "beefy, but muscular, mustachioed" (Leonard et al., 2012, p. 108). All of that vanishes with age. The body exposes weakness, idleness, and lots of wrinkles. In a twist of fate, the gay male body, already feminized by homophobia, is again demasculinized in old age.

Regardless of sexual orientation, the male body is feminized in old age (Thompson, 1994). The attributes of the female body in our gendered system equal those of the old: weak, frail, and home-bound, and experiencing an uncontrolled release of body fluids (Calasanti & King, 2005; Slevin 2008; Slevin et al., 2010). The consumerist culture then offers the means for men to restore their manhood. Men are invited to play and stay hard (to paraphrase Calasanti and King [2005]). What this does is to reaffirm the gender binary and the superiority of masculinity in old age, keeping homosexuality as a different entity, with the consent of the dominant gay male culture (Higgs & McGowan, 2012).

Much of what is demanded by successful aging and the gay culture is attainable only by the middle class. Of course, this might seem obvious, because these demands were created by the white, middle and upper social classes (Slevin, 2008). Likewise, not all gay men have internalized these notions of masculinity and the body, which are reflected in the life stories I collected. Although many of the men I talked to speak about their attempts to age successfully (e.g., exercising, dieting), they also express difficulties in even making ends meet, let alone planning "healthy" meals and exercising. Others struggle with lipodystrophy (body fat redistribution). Similarly, countercultures such as the Radical Faeries, bears, bare-backers, and silver daddies (see Silverdaddies.com and Daddyhunt.com) are defying hegemonic ideas about health, the body, and manhood.

Coupledom

Being single is one of the most significant regrets of Gayby Boomers. When I ask what they would change in their lives or what the least satisfactory aspects of their realities are, the overwhelming response is being single. They lament not working hard enough to date and develop a long-term relationship. They feel alone and unrealized. These feelings of loneliness and failure are the outcome of our prevailing ideology that places the couple as the organizing principle of our lives and the locus of happiness.

Coupledom and marriage are two pillars of heterosexuality (Budgeon, 2008; Sandberg, 2008). We consider them essential for (monogamous) intimacy, sexuality, reproduction, personal development, mutual care, health, support, and financial safety. The couple is everywhere we turn, from Hollywood to the population census, despite demographic trends telling us that more and more people are choosing not to marry. We weep at weddings; students cry from emotion when we show them documentaries about gay nuptials. The couple became the zenith of the gay movement and a gateway to acceptability. The 12 months after my home state's legalization of same-sex marriages, my husband and I attended seven queer weddings (including our own marriage ceremony). Now we have a burgeoning consumer market for LGBT weddings (e.g., equallywed.com). Gay men want to join the institution once decried as the foundation of patriarchy and homophobia, if only for the financial provisions it provides.

Although coupledom is largely a sentimental myth, it is also a reality; it constitutes the basis of our current mode of production and welfare state. Our basic needs are privatized in the family (Fineman, 1995). Spouses and young siblings are supposed to provide care and support for the ill and the elderly (Knauer, 2011). As Fineman explains: "Dependency, 'naturally' assigned to the family, is privatized. It is not anticipated in the ideology that either the market or the state will directly contribute to or assist in the necessary caretaking that is done in the privacy of the family. The ideology of the private family mandates that the unit nurture its members and provide for them economically" (p. 2187).

There is a good amount of shame to being single. "Individuals who are not conventionally coupled often find themselves having to account for their status as though being uncoupled was a deeply problematic condition" (Budgeon, 2008, p. 308). Single (and older) gay men are thought of as emotionally hopeless, egoistic, immature, and lonely. There is also no room for a trio or polyamorous affairs. Coupledom and marriage police monogamy and "proper" sexual relations across age (Sandberg, 2008). Alternatives are few, but single people could think of themselves as independent and achieving (Budgeon, 2008); also, gay men's liaisons such as friends and fuck buddies may support and offer a fulfilling resistance.

The Remains of AIDS

I met Jack, a 62-year-old man, at a drop-in group for LGBT seniors. The afternoon I first saw him, he walked into the room with a cane, yet looked strong—a tall, solid body frame. As I listened to him, I caught a little sense of humor in his speech. He shared his story with the group. Jack is living with HIV and had an AIDS diagnosis more than 20 years ago. Neuropathy causes a constant pain in his feet. He recently moved to the city into a nursing home, after living in the rural Midwest for the past few years. He now plans to move to the YMCA and leave the nursing home. Jack can't stay there longer. He complains of being treated as if he was a "drug addict" and in need of assistance. The staff wants to control his HIV meds. They took all his pills away as instructed by the staff physician, but Jack wants to take the meds as his outside doctor has prescribed. The case manager at the LGBT center is helping him transition to the YMCA.

The next week, Jack sat across from me during our weekly drop-in group. He was restless, grimacing, and rubbing his belly, as if he had abdominal pain. The case manager then walked into the room with a papaya, handed it to Jack, and helped him cut through it in a hurry. With only plastic utensils to do the cutting, Jack's agony was increasing. He ate the chunks of papaya hastily, devouring them. We all observed curiously. Shortly thereafter, and with a regained calm, Jack told us that the HIV meds give him great intestinal discomfort and papaya is the only remedy that soothes the pain.

Jack is a former gay porn star, I learned later. Some guys in the group checked out his movies. They joked with him using sexual innuendos about how "hung" and "good" he was. Jack would talk, nonstop, about any topic, but especially sex. He did not last long in the group. There was an altercation with another group member regarding his sex talk, and that was the last time I saw Jack. He sent a letter to the group via his case manager apologizing and objecting to being wronged and misunderstood by some group members.

Jack did not follow the moral script of an AIDS survivor—acknowledging personal responsibility of his condition. In public forums and popular media, people living with HIV (and or AIDS) usually talk about the careless life they lived and how HIV turned that around, making them more "responsible" beings (see for example, http://www.grayingofaids.org/). Jack was unapologetic, which amplified the stigma. He was treated differently and frequently as "mentally" unstable by both social services professionals and his own LGBT peers.

Although Jack's case is not very common these days, when we think of HIV as a chronic condition, Gayby Boomers who are aging with HIV are seen as different by others, as belonging to a lesser category of older gay people. The stigma toward people living with HIV is not the same as it was during the 1990s, but HIV is still a mark of moral character. Gay men of Jack's generation carry the weight of HIV since the onset of the epidemic. They face rejection, isolation, and shame (Drummond, 2006; Emlet, 2007). Nowadays, those who sero-convert later in life—say, at the age of 55—are labeled as "foolish," "they knew better" (Schrimshaw & Siegel, 2003). Thus, our current narrative of HIV as a chronic condition, the wide spread stigmatization, and the uncertainty about the future, make it difficult for older gay men living with HIV to construct a positive identity as an older person, a gay man, and a person living with HIV.

The consequences of HIV must be analyzed in the context of the life course—timing and transitions (Robinson, Petty, Patton & Kang, 2010). Older men infected with HIV could be living with the virus for decades. Some of them might have sero-converted before the arrival of ARTs, when the virus was equated with death, and were exposed to very toxic medications. Others could have acquired HIV after ARTs. Likewise, some might have gotten HIV at a young age. Young people during the 1980s and 1990s had a whole life to look forward to. These days, young people can go on with their lives with HIV. Older persons might be satisfied with their life and be skillful in managing adversity, and now, in 2015, they face a more certain and less-threatening future. The infection does not alter much of their life course, although they still face some anxiety (Robinson et al., 2010).

Long-term survivors struggle to make sense of their life. During the 1980s and early 1990s, they thought their life was to end prematurely. That changed in 1996 (when ARTs were first used to treat HIV), and the prospect of a longer life increased. Long-term survivors have endured major disruptions in their "imagined life trajectories" (Owen & Catalan,

2012), along with the long-term effects of HIV and the medications. They could have a precarious financial life because they were forced out of the labor market, and some might be unable to work (Owen & Catalan, 2012; Wallach & Brotman, 2013). A couple of men, whose stories you will read here, are on public assistance and do odd jobs (e.g., gardening, cleaning) to make ends meet. They have not recovered financially from losing their job during the 1990s. In addition, gay men of the Baby Boomer generation saw their social networks shrink. If we think of how many of our gay friends came from sexual relationships, then we can appreciate the difficulty of creating new social bonds with gay men when opportunities for sex fall because of HIV and age (Owen & Catalan, 2012).

The epidemic altered the lives and the aging course of Gayby Boomers. Many gay men died prematurely; countless were expected and resigned to die at a young age; some lost their job and family; and most witnessed the loss, guilt, shame, and transformation of youthful physiques into frail, wasted, and uncontrollable bodies—those we associate with old age (Brown, Sarosy, Cook, & Quarto, 1997; Drummond, 2006). Some of the men I talked to speak about "summer funerals," saving their address books to remember lost friendships, and the "over-the-top" drag or disco-themed commemorations. They also express feelings of guilt—the very familiar "why not me?" They think of themselves as survivors: "I feel I am the one who has been left to turn the light out at the end of the party" (Owen and Catalan, 2012, p. 70).

"It would be reasonable to say that virtually every gay person in their later and middle years alive today has been touched by the AIDS epidemic in one form or another through personal illness, infection, loss, and/or caring for those sick from AIDS" (Gorman & Nelson, 2004, p. 79; quoted in Rosenfeld, Bartlam, & Smith, 2012, p. 5). The face of HIV, however, has changed in poignant ways during the past 25 years. Black and Latino populations are now more affected by the epidemic than whites. In addition, a large number of people living with HIV are aging. In the near future, about half of the people living with HIV will be 50 years of age and older (France, 2009). It is not possible to study current gerontology without writing about AIDS.

Today, I find two opposing pulls in our gay culture: one that wants to hold on to the memories and another that wishes to disremember. Gay men in the first group want to keep their history of AIDS alive, either by retelling it or preserving it privately as a part of their individual and collective identities.

I came across Jim at a conference where he was tending an LGBT booth. In my eyes, he looked to be in his mid to late 50s. I had just bought the book *The AIDS Generation* (Halkitis, 2013)—which tells the stories of gay men surviving AIDS—and showed it to him as a conversation motif.

"I probably won't read it." He shrugged his shoulders and looked at to me while holding the book in his hands.

"Have you seen the documentary *We Were Here* (Weissman & Weber, 2011)?" I insist.

"No, I'm not interested."

Then, I begin to empathize. "My partner is the same way; he doesn't watch movies or read books of the AIDS era."

Jim was not interested in the book; I understood it when he told me he had lived in San Francisco all his adult life, until a few years ago. But then I went on to explain that the documentary *We Were Here* recounts the history of AIDS in the San Francisco Bay Area through the testimonials of the people who witnessed and tackled the plague. He had no interest in seeing the film.

"Why?" I asked.

"Because I was there and I don't want to go back there."

My then partner (and now husband), who came of age in New Orleans during the early days of the crisis and voluntarily staffed an AIDS hotline and watched many friends die, feels the same.

Jim does not want his story (if there is one to be told about the plague) to be recounted, hence packaged. I am sure he carries painful memories with him—and a few moments of joy from those years in San Francisco. Grief, shame, guilt, community, love, fear, and resentment. The retelling of his experience, via his own voice or someone else's, might be painful, but also it might domesticate it, which is a dangerous prospect.

But, Jim's response can also speak to the way he has coped. Perhaps he has been able to survive, move to another city, and restart a life by means of locking out what he witnessed. Ironically, not expressing where he has come from in a way of a tale or a therapeutic account works as self-defense strategy. It is a way to preserve who he is and not to be robbed by storytellers like myself.

Those who have chosen to disremember want to erase the marks of AIDS. The disgrace was too upsetting for them. They have decided to wash it off by normalizing—or better, heterosexualizing—their lives, creating a built and vigorous-looking physique; getting married, and parenting (Crimp, 2002). The recent appearance of preexposure prophylaxis (PrEP) has contributed to forgetting the epidemic. PrEP became the latest buzzword in HIV prevention and treatment in 2012, when the Food and Drug

Administration approved the use of the drug Truvada as a PrEP for HIV-negative people. Soon it became part of virtual identities. Many gay men in Grindr, Adam4Adam, and Manhunt now include in their profiles "on PrEP" either as an invitation not to use condoms during intercourse (e.g., "barebacking") or as an assurance of protection. It is a dramatic shift in the history of the epidemic. It provides gay men an added and powerful means of HIV prevention and a license to enjoy sex without condoms. Yet, PrEP makes us erase the memories of AIDS while deepening the medicalization of sex and disease prevention. This pill, which is pretty close to full HIV prevention, was not even imagined during 1980s and 1990s, when the Gayby Boomers were young and trying to make sense of HIV, AIDS, and their collective history.

Queer Time and Life Course

The life stories of the men in *Queer Aging* disrupt the (heterosexually) normative life course. This life trajectory that we perceive as "natural" takes us from birth to schooling, adolescence, job and career, marriage, reproduction, parenthood, maybe divorce, retirement, and death. Although the Baby Boomer generation has challenged this path, it has not changed its essence. For example, Baby Boomers are shifting the retirement experience and resisting aging (or ideas about older age) through consumption and lifestyle choices—again, successful aging. Yet, the heart of aging successfully is precisely that normative conceptualization of the life course, which rests on a capitalist logic of work and time discipline; time and bodies must be used in a productive manner (Castiglia & Reed, 2011; Thompson, 1967).

Queer time is lived outside the narrative of birth, schooling, marriage, reproduction, child bearing, and retirement (Brown, 2009; Sandberg, 2008). It underlines the social construction of time and age as based on biological reproduction (Binnie & Klesse, 2012). The lives of the men I talked to, as well as those documented by other scholars, signal differences in rhythm, paths, and junctures across and within generations (Herdt et al., 1997). Some of them were married heterosexually, have children, and have adopted a gay identity later in their lives. For many, "coming out" and the HIV epidemic were their major life transitions; others have had several romantic relationships and cohabitated with partners, and a few have even entered in same-sex marriages.

The departures from timing and meaning of life events are evident in popular culture and gay literature. In *Beginners* (Urdang et al., and Mills, 2010), the central character, a 75-year-old widower, announces to his son that he is gay, and then goes on to develop a romantic relationship with a much younger man. In 2011, Rick Welts, 58, president of the professional basketball team the Phoenix Suns, came out as a gay man. The story was featured in the *New York Times* (Barty, 2011) and National Public Radio (Siegel, 2011). Welts' story is that of a gay man who kept his sexuality out of the public eye. Only a small circle of friends and family members knew, although there were always rumors within his industry that he was gay. Likewise, very few people knew that his longtime partner died of complications from HIV in 1994, when Welts was 41 years old.

Another insightful example on the timing and meaning of old age in gay men's lives comes from Italian writer Pier Vittorio Tondelli's novel *Separate Rooms* (1989/1992). As I indicated earlier, aging is, arguably, accelerated in gay spaces; scholars have claimed that gay men become "old" during their late 30s (Drummond 2006; Jones & Pugh, 2005). Tondelli, who died in 1991 at the age of 36 from AIDS-related causes, alludes to the queer condition through Leo, the main character in the novel. Leo, a "gay" man (he is not labeled as such in the text), wonders about not being young anymore at the age of 32. Tondelli communicates Leo's thoughts as Leo meditates sitting in a plane looking at his image reflected by the window:

> He still thought of himself and saw himself as an innocent, someone incapable of doing ill or going astray. But the image he saw against that illumined backdrop was simply the face of someone no longer as young as he used to be: someone with fine, thinning hair, puffy eyes, full and slightly flabby lips, and the skin of the cheeks flecked with fine veins, just like his father's livid cheeks. All in all a face of suffering, like any other, the deterioration and the marks of time. He turned thirty-two a few months back. He is well aware that he is not of an age ordinary defined as mature, or even less old. But he also knows that is not young anymore (Tondelli, 1989, pp. 1–2).

This critique of the normative life course and definition of old age comes also from critical gerontologists (Katz and Marshall, 2003; Wallach & Brotman, 2013). Life trajectories are fashioned and sustained by institutions such as education, family, and healthcare, and by the labor and consumer markets. When seen outside such contexts, the differences across chronological age categories and life stages are imprecise. Gay men (and heterosexual persons) then, distance, embrace, and/or negotiate their meanings of age and being old with those of social institutions and gay culture. Their lives, nonetheless, upset governing notions of life course.

The life course perspective invites us to approach the lives of older gay men as relationships among timing, interdependence of lives, and human agency. Life course, as a concept, indicates the interrelation between "age-graded trajectories" (such as careers and intimate relationships) and transitions—say, moving, divorce, and retirement (Elder, 1994, p. 5).

We need to see gay men, not as isolates, but as members of a collective living through particular historical time, undergoing social and political changes, and making life choices within those circumstances—what scholars call *cohorts* (Elder, 1994; Rosenfeld et al., 2012). The approach might be seen as in conflict with queer theory because of its reliance on linear time and sequence, yet we can bracket these assumptions and focus on the interplay of history, social change, and biography, and acknowledge the divergences—within and outside the normative life course (Binnie & Klesse, 2012; Brown, 2009; Kertzner, 2001).

The concept of "generational narratives" proposed by Plummer (2010) bridges the life course perspective and queer theory, helping us read the stories of Gayby Boomers. This notion assumes that lives and sexuality are anchored on age, place, and time. "[T]he stories we tell of social life are usually bound up with the generations we live in—we tell generational narratives" (Plummer, 2010, p. 171). Generations, like cohorts, represent a shared experience (e.g., civil rights movement, AIDS) and worldview—a "fate." But these generational narratives are not identical; they are mediated by social class, race, and nation (Binnie & Klesse, 2012; Plummer, 2010).

In Figure 1.1, I situate the lives of the men in *Queer Aging* by relying on Plummer's (2010) generational narratives. He

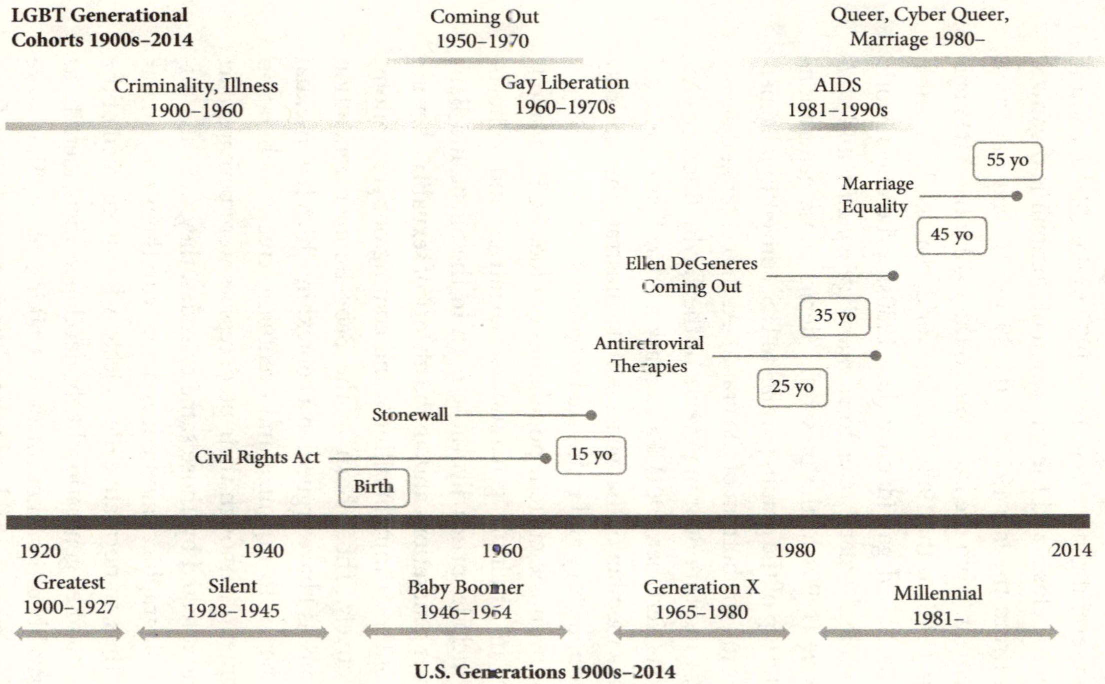

FIGURE 1.1 The lesbian, gay, bisexual, and transgender (LGBT) generational cohorts embedded within the main U.S. generations from the 1900s to 2014 and key historical events. The age across time illustrates the chronological age of a man typical in *Queer Aging* (born in 1956, Baby Boomer generation). Adapted from Plummer (2010).

sketches seven generations in the history of LGBT people in the West: homosexuality as a criminal act and illness (it includes several generations, from 1900 to the 1960s); coming out of the closet and the formation of homophile organizations (from the late 1950s to the 1970s); the gay liberation movement (from the late 1960s to the 1970s); the AIDS epidemic (1981 to the 1990s); queer world, marked by a stable or normalized gay identity (late 1980s); cyberqueer world (1990s); and what I refer to as *marriage equality and childrearing* (1990s to the present). I depict those generations (on the top of the graph) parallel to U.S. conventional generations (on the bottom of the graph). At the center and across time, I indicate defining events of the Gayby Boomer generation (Kertzner, 2001). I also mark a typical chronological age of a member of that generation to illustrate the interplay between history and individual biography.

Within the current population of older LGBT persons there are multiple generational narratives and cohorts; they include, primarily, those born in the Silent and Baby Boomer generations and, in the history of sexuality, they are part of the criminality/illness and coming out generations, respectively. Those born in the Baby Boomer generation grew up, as I have argued, in a context in which homosexual men began to organize and eventually create a liberation movement. Although their predecessors were perhaps part of, and affected by, those same episodes, they were at a different biographical moment and had with them a dissimilar past. Thus, in normative life trajectory language, men of the Baby Boomer generation likely developed their identity as the gay liberation movement was taking place. They were the first ones to think of themselves as gay, different from heterosexual males.

Gayby Boomers, likewise, were the most affected by the AIDS epidemic. They witnessed the highest number of deaths related to AIDS, between 1987 and 1996 (Rosenfeld et al., 2012). Within that time, those age 35 to 44 years had the highest mortality rate than any other group. This, again, shook their individual and collective identities, social networks, sense of community, and aging process. At the personal level, HIV triggered biographical disruptions (Wallach & Brotman, 2013). First, as a terminal condition and, later, as a chronic illness, HIV altered social relations, employment, and routines.

In the same way that Gayby Boomers are a subcohort of the Baby Boomer generation, there are several subcohorts within the former. Those living with HIV constitute a subcohort, and within this group, we have at least two other cohorts, those who acquired HIV before the use of ART and those who did after. Rosenfeld (1999) uses the term *identity cohorts* to capture the subcultures or subgroups within a generation. We can think Gayby Boomers who live with HIV as an identity cohort—with a unique and shared worldview. There are others who "joined" the gay identity at various times and ages. This creates disparities in experience and narratives. For example, it is not the same to come out at the age of 60 in 2011 than at the age of 20 in the 1971 (Rosenfeld, 1999). And of course, there are identity cohorts defined by race, ethnicity, and nation within the Gayby Boomers to which I do not make justice in Figure 1.1, given our limited research of those intersections (Binnie & Klesse, 2012). Nonetheless, the stories of the men in *Queer Aging* hint at the existence of such cohorts, emphasizing the diversity within the generation and the fissures of the normative life course.

As there are departures within generations, there are dialogues and clashes across cohorts. The current experiences of Gayby Boomers are informed by the coexisting generations—men of the criminality/illness, AIDS, and cyber queer worlds (Plummer, 2012). The ongoing changes in the aging of older LGBT people as well as our appreciation of them are influenced not only by Gayby Boomers, but also by synchronal generations. Furthermore, although I have drawn a distinction between queer time and normative life course, I recognize the ambiguity. Not all Gayby Boomers live outside the established heterosexual time regulated by reproduction and capitalism. In the same way, subgroups of heterosexual Baby Boomers have rejected the ideas of reproduction, marriage, and family (Binnie & Klesse, 2012).

Life Stories and Memories

At the heart of *Queer Aging* are the life stories of older gay men. I chose this methodology because I want to grasp the subjective experiences of men—"the inside of aging" (Kenyon, Ruth, & Mader, 1999, p. 54; quoted in Katz, 2000, p. 144), but not in the psychological way. Rather, I see the narratives from a sociological perspective, as they are created within social, cultural, and historical contexts. I do not view accounts as providing information, "facts," or an essence of a person. A story or narrative is an interpretative discourse by which we communicate events, states, and processes while constructing a sense of self and the world (Atkinson, 1998; Hinchman & Hinchman, 1997; Riessman, 1993). They are circumscribed by social norms and a shared language. Here lays the value of narratives: they inform the language available to these men to understand who they are and how they act in the world, as much as language reflects and creates the sociocultural arrangements of their time (Denzin, 1989; Somers, 1992).

But there is also human interest in the stories we tell. They convey emotions, relationships, characters, places, and moments to which many of us sympathize, regardless of our age, gender, or sexual orientation. This is why I present the narratives as standalone cases—for you to connect in a direct manner with the voices of these men. I'm not claiming these are the "true" voices of older gay men, free of any analysis. They are not. These men and I constructed these stories through an interview (Rosenfeld, 1999). I had an agenda, a topic I wanted to learn about. I recruited the men and created an interview protocol. I adjusted my lenses and my questions as I learned from the men through my fieldwork, but I was the one directing this project. Yet, I trust you will relate to these men in the same way I did. And, if not concurring with the conclusions I have drawn, at least taking the stories and deriving your own analysis.

My use of life histories is not only a methodological choice, it is also a theoretical one. It is based on the queer notion of memory as a counteractivity to disremembering. As Castiglia and Reed (2011) put it, through memories we recover the sense of self amidst the institutional practices of denying, ignoring, and cleansing our past. In the prevailing gay discourse, the past is only a site of illness, death, promiscuity, carelessness, and overindulgences. It needed to be disremembered and replaced with a new cleansed version. It required a generational divide. Although the data I present are not entire life histories, they evoke the pleasure and violence of the clandestine, the shame, the bewilderment, the sadness, and the energy and ecstasy of community while centering on the current aging experience. They are not tales of heroism, resilience, or "homonostalgia" (Wekker, 2009). The best I can say is that they are an ongoing effort to live and make sense of the self (constantly), creating a "synthesis" (Castiglia & Reed, 2011) of the past and the present.

The 11 stories I present emerged from 4 years of traditional ethnographic fieldwork (Hammersley & Atkinson, 1995) I did in Chicago. In 2009, I started doing participant observation (e.g., "hanging out") in social and health services organizations and community groups that provide assistance or programming for older LGBT people. I attended meetings and participated in events; talked with dozens of senior LGBT participants, staff members, and advocates; and reviewed groups and organizations' newsletters and other publications. My intention was to immerse myself in what was going on in the city's LGBT communities around aging. Then, narrowing my interest, I conducted a focus group discussion with older gay men (defined as 55 years and older) and individual in-depth interviews with 11 gay men belonging to the Gayby Boomer generation. The age of the men in the interview group range from 55 to 65 years old (born between 1946 and 1957), except for one, Jimmy, who is 71 (born in 1939). I decided to keep Jimmy in the group because he was the only one I found who was caring for his ailing partner—an experience I wished to capture. I selected the men with the purpose of learning about diverse circumstances. Five of the men are white, five are black, and one is of Mexican descent. Of them, five are living with HIV and three are in a relationship (none of them married). I categorize six of them as having a middle social class life (e.g., own a home, have secured retirement income, and are college educated), two as being in the working class, and three as living in poverty (e.g., receiving public aid, struggling to making ends meet, living in unstable housing).

During the interviews I used the life history method (Atkinson, 1998; Hinchman & Hinchman, 1997) first to learn about the men's past (e.g., childhood, family) and then to focus on their current situation. I analyzed the interviews using the holistic-content and interpretative approaches (Denzin & Lincoln, 1994; Lieblich, Tuval-Mashiach, & Zilber, 1998; Silverman, 1993). I examined each interview independently and as a subcase of a larger group. In an iterative process, I moved from interviews, to published literature, my field notes, theoretical frameworks, and back to the interviews, identifying patterns and themes. I then edited the narratives for clarity and ease of reading. I changed the names of the participants as well as potential identifying information to protect their identities. I chose to present the complete freestanding narratives for you to have direct access (although, filtered by me) to the subjective experiences and the voices of these men. Patrick Johnson exemplifies this use of life stories in *Sweet Tea: Black Gay Men of The South* (2008). The stories in *Queer Aging* are more condensed and concise than Johnson's, to avoid redundancy and to highlight the aging context. Nevertheless, the stories of this group of older gay men are more than individual narratives about old age. They tell us about the intersection of history, biography, and social change.

There is nothing extraordinary about the participants in this book that could suggest bias toward a particular phenomenon—say, mental health, poverty, illness, or social status. Many of them have what we might call a regular life; they watch TV, go to the movies, pray, eat meals alone and a few times with family or friends, work full- or part-time, surf the Internet, play cards, hate Chicago's winter, get colds, take health supplements, and occasionally get blue.

I recruited and selected the men using a variety of strategies, such as listservs for LGBT people, social and health services organizations, community groups (e.g., Prime Timers), and social networks. I only knew one of these men before I started this project. A few of them knew each other, but none were close friends.

Each of the following chapters is devoted to a story. They are not organized in any particular way and they are titled using a fictitious name. In the concluding chapter, I return to the framework of queer gerontology in light of these men's stories. I focus on three interrelated themes: identity, shame, and the friendships of gay men.

REFERENCES

American Geriatrics Society Ethics Committee. (2015). American Geriatrics Society care of lesbian, gay, bisexual, and transgender older adults position statement. *Journal of the American Geriatrics Society, 63*(3), 423–426.

Andersen, L. A., & Prohaska, T. R. (2014). Fostering engagement and independence: Opportunities and challenges for an aging society. *Health Education & Behavior, 41*(1 Suppl), 5S–9S.

Atkinson, R. (1998). *The life story interview.* Thousand Oaks, CA: Sage Publications.

Barry, D. (2011, May 15). A sports executive leaves the safety of his shadow life. *New York Times.* Available: http://www.nytimes.com/2011/05/16/sports/basketball/nba-executive-says-he-is-gay.html

Bennett, J. (2008a, September 17). Aging HIV patients face complicated health issues [Online]. *Newsweek.* Available: http://www.newsweek.com/aging-hiv-patients-face-complicated-health-issues-89175.

Bennett, J. (2008b, September 17). Long invisible, gay seniors seek respect, services [Online]. *Newsweek*. Available: http://www.newsweek.com/long-invisible-gay-seniors-seek-respect-services-89161.

Berger, R. M. (1982). *Gay and gray: The older homosexual man*. Urbana, IL: University of Illinois Press.

Binnie, J., & Klesse, C. (2012). The politics of age, temporality, and intergenerationality on transnational lesbian, gay, bisexual, transgender and queer activist networks. *Sociology*, *47*(3), 580–595.

Brown, M. T. (2009). LGBT aging and rhetorical silence. *Sexuality Research & Social Policy*, *6*(4), 65–78.

Brown, L. B., Sarosy, S. G., Cook, T. C., & Quarto, J. G. (1997). *Gay men and aging*. New York: Garland Publishing.

Budgeon, S. (2008). Couple culture and the production of singleness. *Sexualities*, *11*(3), 301–325.

Calasanti, T., & King, N. (2005). Firming the floppy penis: Age, class and gender relations in the lives of old men. *Men and Masculinities*, *8*(1), 3–23.

Casau, N. C. (2005). Perspective on HIV infection and aging: Emerging research on the horizon. *Clinical Infectious Diseases*, *41*(6), 855–863.

Castiglia, C., & Reed, C. (2011). *If memory serves: Gay men, AIDS, and the promise of the queer past*. Minneapolis, MN: University of Minnesota Press.

Center for Disease Control and Prevention. (2015). *HIV among people aged 50 and over* [Online]. Available: http://www.cdc.gov/hiv/group/age/olderamericans/index.html.

Chauncey, G. (1994). *Gay New York: Gender, urban culture, and the making of the gay male world, 1890–1940*. New York, NY: Basic Books.

Chesney, M. A., Chambers, D. B., Taylor, J. M., & Johnson, L. M. (2003). Social support, distress, and well-being in older men living with HIV infection. *Journal of Acquired Immune Deficiency Syndromes*, *33*(Suppl. 2), S185–S193.

Cooperman, N. A., Arnsten, J. H., & Klein, R. S. (2007). Current sexual activity and risky sexual behavior in older men with or at risk for HIV infection. *AIDS Education and Prevention*, *19*(4), 321–333.

Cronin, A., & King, A. (2010). Power, inequality and identification: Exploring diversity and intersectionality amongst older LGB adults. *Sociology, 44*(5), 876–892.

Crimp, D. (2002). *Melancholia and moralism: Essays on AIDS and queer politics*. Cambridge, MA: MIT Press.

Cruz, M. J. (2003). *Sociological analysis of aging: The gay male perspective*. New York, NY: Harrington Park Press.

D'Augelli, A. R., & Grossman, A. H. (2001). Disclosure of sexual orientation, victimization, and mental health among lesbian, gay, and bisexual older adults. *Journal of Interpersonal Violence, 16*(10), 1008–1027.

D'Augelli, A. R., Grossman, A. H., Hershberger, S. L., & O'Connell, T. S. (2001). Aspects of mental health among older lesbian, gay, and bisexual adults. *Aging & Mental Health*, *5*(2), 149–158.

David, S., & Knight, B. G. (2008). Stress and coping among gay men: Age and ethnic differences. *Psychology and Aging, 23*(1), 62–69.

D'Emilio, J. (1998). *Sexual politics, sexual communities*. Chicago, IL: University of Chicago Press.

D'Emilio, J. (2014). *In a new century: Essays on queer history, politics, and community life*. Madison, WI: University of Wisconsin Press.

Denzin, N. (1989). *Interpretative biography*. Newbury Park, CA: Sage Publications.

Denzin, N. K., & Lincoln, Y. S. (1994). *Handbook of qualitative research*. Thousand Oaks, CA: Sage Publications.

De Vries, B., & Blando, J. A. (2004). The study of gay and lesbian aging: Lessons from social gerontology. In H. Gilbert & B. de Vries (Eds.), *Gay and lesbian aging: Research and future directions* (pp. 3–28). New York, NY: Springer.

De Vries, B., & Hoctel, P. (2006). The family–friends of older gay men and lesbians. In N. Teunis & H. Gilbert (Eds.), *Sexual inequalities and social justice* (pp. 230–249). Berkeley, CA: University of California Press.

Dolcini, M. M., Catania, J. A., Stall, R. D., & Pollack, L. (2003). The HIV epidemic among older men who have sex with men. *Journal of Acquired Immune Deficiency Syndromes, 33*(Suppl. 2), S115–S121.

Drummond, M. (2006). Ageing gay men's bodies. *Gay & Lesbian Issues and Psychology Review*, *2*(2), 60–66.

Effros, B. R., Fletcher, C. V., Gebo, K., Halter, J. B., Hazzard, W. R., Horne, F. M., Huebner, R. E., Janoff, E. N., Justice, A. C., Kuritzkes, D., Nayfield, S. G., Plaeger, S. F., Schmader, K. E., Ashworth, J. R., Campanelli, C., Clayton, C. P., Rada, B., Woolard, N. F., & High, K. P. (2008). Workshop on HIV infection and aging: What is known and future research directions. *Aging and Infectious Diseases*, *47*, 542–553.

Elder, H. G. (1994). Time, human agency, and social change perspectives on life course. *Social Psychology Quarterly*, *57*, 4–15.

Ellies, T. (2009). *A phenomenological study of older gay men in San Francisco within the context of socio-cultural change*. Doctoral dissertation, The Wright Institute.

Emlet, C. A. (2007). Experiences of stigma in older adults living with HIV/AIDS: A mixed-methods analysis. *AIDS Patient Care and STDs*, *21*(10), 740–752.

Emlet, C. A. (2008). Truth and consequences: A qualitative exploration of HIV disclosure in older adults. *AIDS Care*, *20*(6), 710–717.

Estes, C. L. (2001). *Social policy & aging: A critical perspective*. Thousand Oaks, CA: Sage Publications.

Estes, C. L., & Binney, E. A. (1989). The biomedicalization of aging: Dangers and dilemmas. *The Gerontologist*, *29*(5), 587–596.

Fabbre, V. D. (2015). Gender transitions in later life: A queer perspective on successful aging. *The Gerontologist*, *55*(1), 144–153.

Ferguson, R. A. (2004). *Aberration in black: Toward a queer of color critique*. Minneapolis, MN: University of Minnesota Press.

Fineman, M. A. (1995). Masking dependency: The political role of family rhetoric. *Virginia Law Review*, *81*, 2181–2215.

Foucault, M. (1995). *Discipline & punish: The birth of the prison* (2nd ed.). New York, NY: Vintage Books.

Foucault, M. (1998). Technologies of the self. In Paul Rabinow (Ed.), *Ethics: Subjectivity and truth*, vol. 1 (pp. 223–251). New York, NY: The New Press.

France, D. (2009). *Another kind of AIDS crisis* [Online]. Available http://nymag.com/health/features/61740/.

Fredriksen-Goldsen, K. I., Kim, H., Goldsen, J., Hoy-Ellis, C. P., Emlet, C. A., Erosheva, E. A., & Muraco, A. (2013). *LGBT older adults in San Francisco: Health, risks, and resilience: Findings from caring with pride*. Seattle, WA: Institute for Multigenerational Health, University of Washington.

Fredriksen-Goldsen, K. I., Kim, H., Shiu, C., Goldsen, J., & Emlet, C. A. (2015). Successful aging among LGBT older adults: Physical and mental health-related quality of life by age group. *The Gerontologist*, *55*(1), 154–168.

Fredriksen-Goldsen, K. I., & Muraco, A. (2010). Aging and sexual orientation: A 25-year review of the literature. *Research on Aging*, *32*(3), 372–413.

Freeman, E. (2010). *Time binds: Queer temporalities, queer histories*. Durham, NC: Duke University Press.

Friend, R. A. (1990). Older lesbian and gay people: A theory of successful aging. *Journal of Homosexuality*, *20*, 99–118.

Funders for Lesbian and Gay Issues. (2004). *Aging in equity: LGBT elders in America*. New York, NY: Funders for Gay and Lesbian Issues.

Gamson, J., & Moon, D. (2004). The sociology of sexualities: Queer and beyond. *Annual Review of Sociology*, *30*, 47–64.

Gorman, E. M., & Nelson, K. (2004). From a far place: Social and cultural considerations about HIV among midlife and older gay men. In H. Gilbert & B. de Vries (Eds.), *Gay and lesbian aging: Research and future directions* (pp. 73–93). New York, NY: Springer.

Gray, H., & Dressel, P. (1985). Alternative interpretations of aging among gay males. *The Gerontologist*, *25*(1), 83–87.

Green, A. I. (2007). Queer theory and sociology: Locating the subject and the self in sexuality studies. *Sociological Theory*, *25*(1), 26–45.

Green, A. I. (2008). Health and sexual status in an urban gay enclave: An application of the stress process model. *Journal of Health & Social Behavior*, *49*, 436–451.

Gross, J. (2007, October 9). Aging and gay, and facing prejudice in twlight. *New York Times*. Available: http://www.nytimes.com/2007/10/09/us/09aged.html?_r=0

Grossman, A. H. (2008). The unique experiences of older gay and bisexual men: Associations with health and well-being. In R. J. Wolitski, R. Stall, & R. O. Valdiserri (Eds.), *Unequal opportunity: Health disparities affecting gay and bisexual men in the United States* (pp. 303–326). New York, NY: Oxford University Press.

Grossman, A. H., D'Augelli, A. R. D., & Hershberger, S. L. (2000). Social support networks of lesbian, gay, and bisexual adults 60 years of age and older. *Journal of Gerontology: Social Sciences, 55B*, P171–P179.

Hajek, C. (2014). Gay men at midlife: A grounded theory of social identity management through linguistic labeling and intra- and intergenerational talk. *Journal of Language and Social Psychology, 33*(6), 606–631.

Halberstam, J. (2005). In a queer time and place: Transgender bodies, subcultural lives. New York, NY: New York University Press.

Halkitis, P. N. (2013). *The AIDS generation: Stories of survival and resilience*. New York, NY: Oxford University Press.

Hammersley, M., & Atkinson, P. (1995). *Ethnography: Principles in practice*. New York, NY: Routledge.

Hartocollis, A. (2011, August 12). Jacques Beaumont and Richard Townsend. *New York Times*. Available: http://www.nytimes.com/2011/08/14/fashion/weddings/jacques-beaumont-and-richard-townsend-vows.html?pagewanted=all&_r=2.

Heaphy, B. (2007). Sexualities, gender and ageing: Resources and social change. *Current Sociology, 55*(2), 193–210.

Heckman, T. G., Kochman, A., Sikkema, K. J., Kalichman, S. C., Masten, J., & Goodkin, K. (2000). Late middle-aged and older men living with HIV/AIDS: Race differences in coping, social support, and psychological distress. *Journal of the National Medical Association, 92*(9), 436–444.

Herdt, G., Beeler, J., & Rwals, T. W. (1997). Life course diversity among older lesbians and gay men: A study in Chicago. *Journal of Gay, Lesbian, and Bisexual Identity, 2*, 231–246.

Herdt, G., & de Vries, B. (Eds.). (2004). *Gay and lesbian aging: Research and future directions*. New York, NY: Springer.

Higgs, P., & McGowan, F. (2012). Aging, embodiment and the negotiation of third and fourth ages. In A. Kampf, B. L. Marshall, & A. Petersen (Eds.), *Aging men, masculinities and modern medicine* (pp. 21–34). New York, NY: Routledge.

High, K. P., Brennan-Ing, M., Clifford, D. B., Cohen, M. H., Currier, J., Deeks, S. G., Deren, S., Effros, R. B., Gebo, K., Goronzy, J. J., Justice, A. C., Landay, A., Levin, J., Miotti, P. G., Munk, R. J., Nass, H., Rinaldo, C.R.Jr, Shlipak, M. G., Tracy, R., Valcour, V., Vance, D. E., Walston, J. D., Volberding, P. OAR Working Group on HIV and Aging. (2012). HIV and aging: State of knowledge and areas of critical need for research: A report to the NIH Office of AIDS Research by the HIV and Aging Working Group. *Journal of Acquired Immune Deficiency Syndromes*, *60*(Suppl. 1), S1–S18.

Hinchliff, S. (2009). Ageing and sexual health in the UK. *Journal of Health Psychology*, *14*(3), 355–360.

Hinchman, L. P., & Hinchman, S. K. (1997). Introduction. In L. P. Hinchman & S. K. Hinchman (Eds.), *Memory, identity, community: The idea of narrative in the human sciences*. Albany, NY: State University of New York Press.

Hughes, M. (2006). Queer aging. *Gay and Lesbian Issues and Psychology Review*, *2*(2), 54–59.

Institute of Medicine of the National Academies. (2011). *The health of lesbian, gay, bisexual, and transgender people: Building a foundation for better understanding*. Washington, DC: National Academy of Science.

Jackson, N. C., Johnson, M. J., & Roberts, R. (2008). The potential impact of discrimination fears of older gays, lesbians, bisexuals and transgender individuals living in small- to moderate-sized cities on long-term health care. *Journal of Homosexuality*, *54*(3), 325–339.

Jimenez, A. D. (2003). Triple jeopardy: Targeting older men of color who have sex with men. *Journal of Acquired Immune Deficiency Syndromes*, *33*(Suppl. 2), S222–S225.

Johnson, M. J., Jackson, N. C., Arnette, J. K., & Koffman, S. D. (2005). Gay and lesbian perceptions of discrimination in retirement care facilities. *Journal of Homosexuality*, *49*(2), 83–102.

Johnson, P. E. (2008). *Sweet Tea: Black Gay Men of the South.* Chapel Hill: University of North Carolina Press.

Jones, J., & Pugh, S. (2005). Ageing gay men: Lessons from the sociology of embodiment. *Men and Masculinities, 7,* 248–260.

Kahana, E., & Kahana, B. (2001). Successful aging among people with HIV/AIDS. *Journal of Clinical Epidemiology, 54*(Suppl. 1), S53–S56.

Katz, S. (2000). Busy bodies: Activity, aging, and the management of everyday life. *Journal of Aging Studies, 4*(2), 135–152.

Katz, S., & Marshall, B. (2003). New sex for old: Lifestyle, consumerism, and the ethics of aging well. *Journal of Aging Studies, 17*(1), 3–16.

Kayal, P. M. (1994). Communalization and homophile organization membership: Gay volunteerism before and during AIDS. *Journal of Gay and Lesbian Social Services, 1,* 33–57.

Kelly, J. (1977). The aging male homosexual. *The Gerontologist, 17*(4), 328–332.

Kenyon, G. M., Ruth, J., & Mader, W. (1999). Elements of a narrative gerontology. In V. L. Bengtson & K. W. Schaie (Eds.), *Handbook of theories of aging* (pp. 40–58). New York, NY: Springer.

Keppel, B., & Firestein, B. (2007). Bisexual inclusion in addressing issues of GLBT aging: Therapy with older bisexual women and men. In B. Firenstein (Ed.), *Becoming visible: Counseling bisexuals across the lifespan* (pp. 164–185). New York, NY: Columbia University Press.

Kertzner, R. M. (2001). The adult life course and homosexual identity in midlife gay men. *Annual Review of Sexual Research, 12,* 75–92.

Kimmel, D., Rose, T., Orel, N., & Greene, B. (2006). Historical context for research on lesbian, gay, bisexual, and transgender aging. In D. Kimmel, T. Rose, & S. David (Eds.), *Lesbian, gay, bisexual, and transgender aging: Research and clinical perspectives* (pp. 1–19). New York, NY: University of Columbia Press.

Knauer, N. J. (2011). *Gay and lesbian elders: History, law, and identity politics in the United States.* Surrey, BC: Ashgate.

Krehely, J. (2009). *How to close the LGBT health disparities gap: Disparities by race and ethnicity.* Washington, DC.: Center for American Progress.

Kreider, T. (2013, January 20). You are going to die. *New York Times.* Available: http://opinionator.blogs.nytimes.com/2013/01/20/you-are-going-to-die/.

Laws, G. (1993). The land of old age: Society's changing attitudes toward urban built environments for elderly. *Annals of the Association of American Geographers, 83*(4), 672–693.

Leonard, W., Duncan, D., & Barrett, C. (2012). What a difference a gay makes: The construction of the older gay man. In A. Kampf, B. L. Marshall, A. Petersen (Eds.), *Aging men, masculinities and modern medicine* (pp. 105–120). New York, NY: Routledge.

Lewis, N. M. (2009). Mental health in sexual minorities: Recent indicators, trends, and their relationships to place in North America and Europe. *Health & Place, 15,* 1029–1045.

Lieblich, A., Tuval-Mashiach, R., & Zilber, T. (1998). *Narrative research: Reading, analysis, and interpretation.* Thousand Oaks, CA: Sage Publications.

Lovejoy, T. I., Heckman, T. G., Sikkema, K. J., Hansen, N. B., Kochman, A., Suhr, J. A., Garske, J. P., & Johnson, C. J. (2008). Patterns and correlates of sexual activity and condom use behavior in persons 50-plus years of age living with HIV/AIDS. *AIDS and Behavior, 12*(6), 943–956.

Lyons, A., Pitts, M., Grierson, J., Thorpe, R., & Power, J. (2010). Ageing with HIV: Health and psychosocial well-being of older gay men. *AIDS Care, 22*(10), 1236–1244.

Marks, H. (Producer) & Winer, L. (Director). (1985). *Silent Pioners* [Documentary]. United States: Silent Pioneers Productions.

Massad, J. A. (2002). Re-orienting desire: The gay international and the Arab world. *Public Culture, 14*(2), 361–385.

McMahon, E. (2003). The older homosexual: Current concepts of lesbian, gay, bisexual, and transgender older Americans. *Clinics in Geriatric Medicine, 19*(3), 587–593.

MetLife. (2010). *Still out, still aging: The MetLife study of lesbian, gay, bisexual, and transgender baby boomers.* Westport, CT: MetLife Mature Market Institute. Available: https://www.

metlife.com/assets/cao/mmi/publications/studies/2010/mmi-still-out-still-aging.pdf.

MetLife, Lesbian and Gay Aging Issues Network of the American Society of Aging, & Zogby International. (2006). *Out and aging: The MetLife Study of Lesbian and Gay Baby Boomers.* Westport, CT: MetLife Mature Market Institute.

Musick, M. A., & Wilson, J. (2008). *Volunteers: A Social Profile.* Bloomington: Indiana University Press.

National Gay and Lesbian Task Force. (2005). Make room for all: Diversity, cultural competence & discrimination in an aging America. Washington, DC: National Gay and Lesbian Task Force.

Owen, G., & Catalan, J. (2012). "We never expected this to happen": Narratives of ageing with HIV among gay men living in London, UK. *Cult Health Sex, 14*(1), 59–72.

Pew Research Center. (2014). *Millennials in adulthood: Detached from institutions, networked with friends.* Available: http://www.pewsocialtrends.org/2014/03/07/millennials-in-adulthood/.

Plummer, K. (2010). Generational sexualities, subterranean traditions, and the hauntings of the sexual world: Some preliminary remarks. *Symbolic Interaction, 33*(2), 163–190.

Powell, J. L. (2004). Ageing, technologies of self and biomedicine: A Foucauldian excursion. *International Journal of Sociology and Social Policy, 24*(6), 17–29.

Powell, J. L., & Biggs, S. (2003). Foucauldian gerontology: A methodology for understanding aging. *Journal of Sociology.* Available: http://www.sociology.org/content/vol7.2/03_powell_biggs.html.

Quam, J. K., & Whitford, G. S. (1992). Adaptation and age-related expectations of older gay and lesbian adults. *The Gerontologist, 32*(3), 367–374.

Raws, T. W. (2004). Disclosure and depression among older gay and homosexual men: Findings from the Urban Men's Health Study. In H. Gilbert & B. de Vries (Eds.), *Gay and lesbian aging: Research and future directions* (pp. 117–141). New York, NY: Springer.

Riessman, C. K. (1993). *Narrative analysis.* Newbury Park, CA: Sage Publications.

Robinson, W. A., Petty, M. S., Patton, C., & Kang, H. (2010). Aging with HIV: Historical and intra-community differences in experience of aging with HIV. In J. T. Sears (Ed.), *Growing older: Perspective on LGBT aging* (pp. 104–121). New York, NY: Routledge.

Roediger, D. R. (1991). *The wages of whiteness: Race and the making of the American working class*. London: Verso.

Rosenfeld, D. (1999). Identity work among lesbian and gay elderly. *Journal of Aging Studies*, *13*(2), 121–144.

Rosenfeld, D., Bartlam, B., & Smith, R. D. (2012). Out of the closet and into the trenches: Gay male Baby Boomers, aging, and HIV/AIDS. *The Gerontologist*, *52*(2), 255–264.

Rowe, W. J., & Kahn, R. L. (1987). Human Aging: usual and successful. *Sciences*, *237*(4811), 143–149.

SAGE. (n.d. a). *About us: History*. Available: http://www.sageusa.org/about/history.cfm.

SAGE. (n.d. b). *25 Lessons on successful aging*. Available: http://sageusa.org/successfulaging/.

SAGE. (2014). *Out and visible: The experiences and attitudes of lesbian, gay, bisexual, and transgender older adults, ages 45–75*. New York, NY: SAGE.

Sandberg, L. (2008). The old, the ugly and the queer: Thinking old age in relation to queer theory. *Graduate Journal of Social Sciences*, *5*(2), 117–139.

Schrimshaw, E. W., & Siegel, K. (2003). Perceived barriers to social support from family and friends among older adults with HIV/AIDS. *J Health Psychol*, *8*(6), 738–752.

Shippy, R. A., Cantor, M. H., Brennan, M. (2004). Social networks of aging gay men. *Journal of Men's Studies*, *13*, 107–120.

Siegel, R. (2011, May 16). Head of Phoenix Suns says he's gay. *National Public Radio*. Available: http://www.npr.org/2011/05/16/136368712/head-of-phoenix-suns-says-hes-gay

Silverman, D. (1993). *Interpreting qualitative data: Methods for analysing talk, text and interaction*. London: Sage.

Slevin, K. F. (2008). Disciplining bodies: The aging experiences of older heterosexual and gay men. *Generations*, *32*(1), 36–42.

Slevin, K., Thomas, F., & Linneman, J. (2010). Old gay men's bodies and masculinities. *Men and Masculinities*, *12*(4), 483–507.

Somers, M. R. (1992). Special section: Narrative analysis in social sciences, part 2. Narrativity, narrative identity, and social action: Rethinking English working class formation. *Social Science History, 16*(4), 591–630.

Steffens, D. C., Fisher, G. G., Langa, K. M., Potter, G. G., & Plassman, B. L. (2009). Prevalence of depression among older Americans: The Aging, Demographics and Memory Study. *International Psychogeriatrics, 21*(5), 879–888.

Stein, A., & Plummer, K. (1994). "I can't even think straight": "Queer" theory and the missing sexual revolution in sociology. *Sociological Theory, 12*(2), 178–187.

Thompson, E. P. (1967). Time, work-discipline, and industrial capitalism. *Past and Present, 38*, 56–97.

Thompson, E. H. (1994). *Older men's lives.* Thousand Oaks, CA: Sage Publications.

Tondelli, P. V. (1989/1992). *Separate Rooms*. London: Serpent's Tail.

Twigg, J. (2004).The body, gender and age: Feminist insights in social gerontology. *Journal of Aging Studies, 18*, 59–73.

Urdang, L., Vanech, D., de Pencier, M., Knudsen, Hoy, J. V. (Producers) & Mills, M. (Director). (2010). Beginners [Motion Picture]. United States: Olympus Pictures.

Valocchi, S. (2005). Not yet queer enough: The lessons of queer theory for the sociology of gender and sexuality. *Gender and Society, 19*(6), 750–770.

Vance, D. E., McGuinness, T., Musgrove, K., Orel, N. A., & Fazeli, P. L. (2011). Successful aging and the epidemiology of HIV. *Clin Interv Aging, 6*, 181–192.

Wallace, P. S., Cochran, D. S., Durazo, M. E., & Ford, L. C. (2011). *The health of aging lesbian, gay and bisexual adults in California* (p. 8). Los Angeles, CA: University of California Los Angeles.

Wallach, I., & Brotman, S. (2013). Ageing with HIV/AIDS: A scoping study among people aged 50 and over living in Quebec. *Ageing and Society, 33*(7), 1212–1242.

Warner, M. (1999). *The trouble with normal: Sex, politics, and the ethics of queer life*. New York, NY. The Free Press.

Weinstein, S. (2007). Fiction of desire. *Out, 16*(5), 50–53.

Weissman, D., & Weber, B. (2011). *We were here.*

Wekker, G. (2009). Van Homo Nostalgie en Betere Tijden: Multiculturaliteit en Postkolonialiteit [Of gay nostalgia and better times: Multiculturality and postcoloniality]. George Mosse Lecture 2009. Amsterdam.

White, A. M., Philogene, G. S., Fine, L., & Sinha, S. (2009). Social support and self-reported health status of older adults in the United States. *American Journal of Public Health*, *99*(10), 1872–1878.

Wight, R. G., LeBlanc, A. J., de Vries, B., & Detels, R. (2012). Stress and mental health among midlife and older gay-identified men. *American Journal of Public Health*, *102*(3), 503–510.

Willigen, V. M. (2000). Differential benefits of volunteering across the life course. *Journal of Gerontology: Social Sciences*, *55B*, S308–S318.

World Health Organization. (2014). *Facts about ageing.* Available: http://www.who.int/ageing/about/facts/en/.

STAN

"If I'm Left, Then I Have to Be the Best Little Gay Boy Ever"

I WAS BORN IN MARYLAND, in a rural and very isolated area during the 1950s. Growing up there in the '50s was like growing up in the Mississippi Delta during the 1930s—a very backward area. I moved to Chicago in 1978 after getting my PhD, then I went back East (to Washington, DC) in 1984 to work in scientific publications. I was an editor for 2 years. That was also the time when the AIDS crisis was reaching a peak, and I was the editor of AIDS articles for 2 years. Then I moved back to Chicago and I've been here ever since. Now I work for the city of Chicago. I'm 59, have no relatives, and am single. I went to high school in Maryland and left to go to an Ivy college, then I went to a research university for my PhD.

Now I don't have any free time. But before, I enjoyed reading—still do—and writing. Before I took this position I was a long-distance runner. I did a lot of running, and that's actually how I came out officially: through the Front Runners club in Washington, DC. I had been out socially before then, but in 1984, when I moved to Washington, there was a Front Runners organization and I joined it and I really came out sort of officially. Everywhere I've gone since then, I have been involved with Front Runners. I'm still a member. The other thing that I do is needlepoint, which is very tactile. It really relaxes me. And of course I do have friends. I go out with friends and I socialize with them.

The narrowing of possibilities is what I think about as I get older. I don't have as many options as I had before, just because time is limited. Also urgency—there is sort of an urgency to do what I want to do while I'm still here. One of the things that probably comes on both sides of that is the urgency and the lack of time that's left. I think about the things I haven't had, the experiences I haven't had. One of them is that I've never had a partner. Although there is no urgency (I don't feel like I have to have one immediately), it's an experience that I would like to have before I die, having somebody in my life.

I grew up alone. My parents have two children. I have a sister, but she is 13 years younger than I am. There was a child in between, but that child died at birth. I remember really enjoying the activities available to us growing up in Maryland on a farm: the woods, the water, swimming, boating, crabbing. My mother and father did not own the farm, but we lived in the country, and my aunts and uncles all lived on farms. I was always going to their homes on my bicycle—just playing all day long. It was very idyllic. I did a lot of reading when I was a little kid because I was left alone a lot. Both of my parents worked, so after I was old enough to stay by myself in the house, they would leave me. My grandparents lived next door, in case there was an emergency. We had 5 acres of land; our two houses were close together and then the land was all around us.

It was just my life. The town was small—just 350 people—and as a group of children we were pretty much allowed to run into town. There seemed to be older people and children, and nobody in between. They were probably gone, working. During some hot summer days when we were off from school, the kids would all get together on their bicycles and we would just range all over. We played in the woods, we had tree houses, we played down at the river, we had boathouses, and we went down to the boats. It was a really neat way to grow up.

We were poor. We didn't have a lot of money. My parents never made more than $10,000 a year, but we didn't know we were poor. We grew our own vegetables. The entire family chipped in together and we bought a cow. Every year we slaughtered the bull and ate the beef. One of my uncles would raise the bull. We had a butchering day; we had to go down to his farm and butcher the cow. We also had the seafood from the river. We had fresh fish, fresh crab—all of that we caught ourselves—and when we caught enough, we would freeze the rest. I didn't grow up feeling like I was poor. In fact, I grew up thinking I was rich, because there were all these wealthy families around us. We all knew one another, and everybody needed one another in a small town; it was so isolated and everybody pitched in.

Social class was based on who you were and your family. You could be poor as a church mouse, but if you came from a good family, you were fine, and you were always welcome in other people's homes. You were always part of the social structure. It was different, much different than here now.

My mother and father were in a mixed marriage. My mother was Catholic and my father was Episcopalian. They could not be married in the Church; they were married on my aunt's farm. The agreement was that I would be raised Catholic. I was brought up Catholic, with all of the structures the Catholic Church puts on you. My mother took all of it with a grain of salt; she wasn't the most indoctrinating person. My favorite memory is that we went to church one Sunday and the priest gave a long sermon on birth control. We then went to breakfast and we were sitting there at the breakfast table when my mother looked at me, and she said, "You don't believe everything the priest tells you, do you?"

And I said, "Not everything."

"I want you to know that if your father and I didn't practice birth control, then we would have many more children and we would be very poor." Her argument was to take the overall message, but you didn't have to live with the specifics.

My father was busy at work, but he was not very personal. He was not very fatherly; he was very distant.

I was a sickly child. I had asthma and I had pneumonia and a whole bunch of things when I was little. The doctors made me eat. They gave me medicine and made me eat. So I gained weight; I had been very frail. I became sort of a hefty boy, which is what I am now—back to being that, unfortunately. I was a hefty boy and I was not good at sports, and there was a class issue about sports. My mother didn't really want me associating with the boys who were in town and on the baseball team because they were sort of the rough boys, not of our class. My mother was not really eager to see me with the other boys because she felt they were trouble. In many cases, they were. So I had these really isolated teenage years.

It was also very clear that I had to go to college to get out of there. There were no jobs. It was all based on farming and fishing. I wasn't going to do any of that. I had to go to college and get the heck out of there. That meant that I studied all the time because there was no money, so I had to get a scholarship.

I knew there was no place for me. I knew I was different. Everybody knew I was different. I was teased a lot there because I was different from everybody else. Nobody really could put their finger on it. I was never accused of being gay or any of that, but everybody knew I was different, and I did too and I knew I had to leave. I just looked at the world differently. I wanted to be part of a greater part of the world. I didn't want to be isolated in this little pocket.

I was a choir boy and an altar boy. When I was in my later teens, 16 to 17, I became a lector. I was very much a part of the church structure in the town. In fact, when I left, my priest, who was a Jesuit, gave me a Bible, which I still have. I enjoyed doing what I was doing. I didn't think I had a vocation and I wasn't enamored with the Church; it was just something you'd do. It was the social structure in town and I had been going there since I was born.

I went to a private college—a second tier of the Ivy League—and I was on a full scholarship. Suddenly, I was in college with kids from New York, New Jersey, Connecticut, and all of whose parents were lawyers and doctors. I saw life from a different point of view. I saw how conservative it was where I came from, because this was the '60s, after all, and the '60s sort of passed me by.

I really think getting my degree and coming out were the two most important things that happened to me. I didn't come out until I was 28, but I struggled with it in graduate school a great deal. As pretty much could be predicted, I fell in love with my roommate. I had to deal with that. Then I started experimenting in the university town. The last couple of years I was in graduate school I would sneak off to the movie house in the city just to see people, just to figure out. It wasn't very nice. I didn't really come out until after I got my PhD and moved to Chicago. Within a couple of months, I got the courage to call a gay hotline. I was directed to go to Halsted Street and I sort of made my way down there in the middle of winter. I just stood and looked. Everybody was like, "Oh, oh, so this is what it is all about."1979. The bar I went to was The Bushes.

Then I went to Washington, and the first papers identifying the virus were sitting on a desk next to mine at the editorial house I was working for. We were just about to publish them. I was working on those and helping people with other papers about HIV/AIDS. Then, I realized what has happening and I called a former boyfriend of mine who I knew was ill. I said, "Do you have AIDS? You need to tell me now." We were sexually active. "I was your last boyfriend; we need to have this conversation." He broke down on the phone and he said, yes, he had the gay disease and he was dying. We both cried for a while. He died soon after that.

I worked for the scientific journal of record for HIV/AIDS research in America. We had a rush to publish policy; we knew how important it was. For those 2 years, I was one of the world's experts on the epidemiology of AIDS because I reviewed all the articles that were being submitted to the magazine. I didn't do the research, but I saw everything way ahead of time.

As I mentioned, I had joined Front Runners and, one by one, people started to get the disease. The president, who was a strapping and unbelievably handsome attorney and a great runner, disappeared. We didn't know what happened to him. I was walking down the street a couple of months later and here was this old, bent, crippled man walking toward me. I realized it was him. I was like, "Oh shit." So my friends were dropping sort of one by one all around me. It was really horrible, because there wasn't anything you could do.

I knew more about AIDS research than anybody else in the city. I suddenly was on a dinner circuit; people were inviting me to have dinner with people who had HIV or AIDS. I was invited for two reasons. I was invited to be the buffer between those who didn't have it and those who did have it, because everybody who didn't have it was scared. They were scared of the guests who did have it. I was the guest who was seated between the people who didn't have it and the ones who had it. I wasn't afraid of them. I knew what it was; I knew how it spread. The other reason why I was invited to dinner was that the AIDS patients wanted to ask me what was going on with AIDS research.

I lost a lot of friends during that time. I lost a whole group of friends. One by one, they all died. That was really sad. There are only a couple of them left. So, that made me cautious about sex and sexual relations, but at the same time, I wasn't being particularly safe. I mean, my attitude was, "If I'm going to get it, I'm going to get it." I was sexually active in the '80s, in Washington. I'm versatile in terms of what I do; I could have contracted it several ways, but I never did.

I think I have immunity to AIDS, because there is another disease that I never got—measles, the really bad kind. When I was a child the whole school got it. We had a three-room school house, six grades in three rooms, and everyone got the measles. I never got the measles. The doctors where all kind of amazed.

I had an affair with a guy in San Francisco that was quite wild, and we had a wonderful time and we still are friends. He developed HIV; I didn't. He is still living; his cell count never went down. But, he called me up after our relationship ended and he said, "I've developed it and you need to go get tested."

I said, "No, I've been tested and I'm HIV negative."

I felt like I was in a war; I was like a war survivor. I have survivor syndrome. I had it and suffered from it for a long time. It was hard: "Why them and not me?" Then there is part of it that is: "If I'm left, then I have to be the best little gay boy ever." If I didn't get it, and I'm left, and I have to represent the entire community, I have to be the best gay person I can possibly be, because I'm going to be the worst nightmare the religious Right has ever had.

I had to work really hard to represent all those people who died. I was on the frontlines when Reagan wouldn't even talk about it. One of my friends from college was writing all Reagan's speeches and Reagan wouldn't even use the words *HIV* or *AIDS* in his speeches. I was furious. It made me very angry and very determined to do something and to represent those who had died and to be the best I could possibly be. At the same time, it made me feel guilty that I had survived and they hadn't. As I said, I had survivor's guilt.

My Southern upbringing helped me deal with the adversity, because there's been adversity from the very beginning, and you just lift up your skirts and go. Tomorrow is another day. You just push on through and that's what you do—very Scarlet O'Hara. I think that's what helped me deal with adversity: the examples of my mother and my grandmothers dealing with it; the pride that they had, not in the best way, in themselves and in what they were doing; the fact that no matter how little money we had, but who we were as people. I'm not so sure how the survivor's guilt affected everything. I'm not that self-aware. I know I have the guilt. I know it's made me fearful, a little bit. I just don't know the answer to how it changed me.

The idea of Front Runners is to be a positive example of gay life in the community. One of its purposes is to bring people together and, certainly in the '80s, that was very important—to bring people together with common interests and build comradeship by sharing those interests and participating in races and going out running together. When you run with people, you bond with them; that was the idea of a runners club. The other part of Front Runners is to be a positive example in the community of the gay life. It's very healthy; it's about doing for others. For example, we do water stations for marathons and for other races.

The best example of why this is effective came from a woman out in Wisconsin. She was part of a running club there and she came up to me one time and she said, "You know what? We have a lot of fun in our running club, but you guys, you have a lot of fun, but you also stand for something." That message has been very clear—that we are there to help them as much as we are to help ourselves.

When I went back to Chicago, I joined Front Runners there. This was after having belonged in Washington. I worked myself up from being secretary to president. The year of my presidency, the now-former CEO of AIDS Walk, which went belly-up, became very homophobic. Front Runners was one of the organizations that had been there since the beginning to help the AIDS Walk every year. The executive director of AIDS Walk didn't want anybody with gay-identifiable clothing volunteering. She was afraid. "It would scare away our corporate funding," she said. She banned Front Runners from helping and participating. She also banned family members of AIDS victims, because she was afraid that would offend the corporate sponsors. *Are you fucking kidding me?* I met with other activists. I spread the word about what was happening, and AIDS Walk started getting a lot of flack over it. People were calling, saying, "What the heck?"

I decided that, as a good gay boy and as a good Chicagoan, I knew what talked in that town. We were not going to boycott the walk; we were going to participate and we were going to raise more money than anybody else. Front Runners joined the AIDS Walk. We signed up to march instead of volunteering. I encouraged everybody in the club to raise as much money as they could. I went to every single attorney I knew and said, "Pony up." I collected more money than anybody else and I put it together with the club's money. I got the money all in cash, and I went to the head of the AIDS Walk board; I didn't go to the AIDS Walk people.

I gave her the cash and I said, "I want a receipt for this now. Here is my donation from the club. I want you to count it, I want a receipt for it, and then we'll talk."

She gave me the receipt and asked, "What do you want?"

I said, "I want to meet with you tomorrow morning at breakfast. We are going to have breakfast or I'm going to go to the papers."

She called me that afternoon and asked, "What do I need to bring to breakfast?"

I said, "I want a list of all your contributors by zip code. You can generate that overnight."

So she brought the list. Front Runners' zip code, 60657 (Lakeview, also known as "Boystown"), had contributed more money than anybody else. I stripped every corporate donation.

"Give me a break!" I said. "You are working against the people that are giving you the money." It was a success, but I was pissed.

Front Runners has given me self-esteem and focus. It opened up worlds to me. As I mentioned, was a very unathletic boy. I never had this view of myself as an athlete. Front Runners gave me the self-confidence not only to be as good a runner as I could be, but also I did four marathons with them. I've met people around the world. Plus, it's given me lots of role models. Front Runners has saved my life.

I don't have a lot of friends. I have a couple of people that I can talk to and socialize with on a regular basis, but there is nobody to really support me. At least I don't see it that way. I'm in therapy. In the late 1990s, when I went to work in a small town on the East Coast, I suddenly felt lost, totally disconnected. I didn't know anybody there and I was living in a situation where I would get up in the morning in the dark, at 4:00 or 4:30 in the morning, I would drive to work, and I would be in an isolated research center that had acres of land around it, to make it isolated quite deliberately. Then, I would drive home at night, I would stop at the gym, but people were very unfriendly, and I would go home. I never saw anybody in the apartment complex I lived in. There were no sidewalks. I had a breakdown pretty quickly—a pretty serious one.

When I moved back to Chicago and had a relapse of the breakdown, I went under treatment right away. I took Paxil and that put a floor under me. I was able to function. I started therapy, and that has really helped see the need to connect to people, and it sort of brought me back to a point where I could. I think, just looking at it as a process, the breakdown came because of years of dealing with all kinds of stuff—being gay being one of them. Therapy has really helped me become human again. It was sort of like the breakdown was necessary and I've rearranged the pieces and the pieces have come back better.

I think the gay community only sees gay men as being between 27 and 40. That's their image of what gay men are. I don't think they even register there are older gay people with different kinds of lives. My generation of gay men, who are aging, are going to be the people who define it. The generation before us was dealing with the AIDS crisis, and there are so few of them, relatively, that they've been dealing with the AIDS crisis and the aftermath of that in their lives more than with how to define being older in the gay community. My generation and the ones coming after me have more people left. My generation probably lost a lot of people, but the ones of us who are left are sort of defining what it means to be older because we are out. We are trying to figure out what it means to be an older gay man.

I pity the gay men who are not modifying their behavior, from when they were in their 20s and 40s, and who still behave in a very postadolescent way as gay men in their late 60s. I see them being frustrated and lonely, not really knowing how to act, because they are not the center of attention anymore. They are not the pretty young things; they're not the drop-dead gorgeous gay guys. You need to modify your behavior to where you are in your life. This doesn't mean that you give up things; it means that you get greater and greater depth as you go along, that you should be digging deeper and developing yourself deeper. No longer should you be on the surface.

My health is not great. My doctor thinks I have diabetes. I had two pulmonary embolisms—one in the mid '90s and one in 2002—then I gained a lot of weight. My disappointment with my doctor is a matter of his style. I think it's a style that all physicians are coming to: he sits in the room and clocks on the computer while you talk to him, and it's all based on what's on the computer and not on his skill. My previous doctor never made a notation. I mean he would write something, once in a while, but it was more of sitting there and him examining me.

There are parts of my life that haven't been developed. One of those, which I mentioned earlier, is that I never had a partnership. I haven't dated in over 10 years, which is sad, but it's also a function of being in public affairs profession. It's hard to date anybody when you are at work 12 hours a day.

I'm not a very spiritual person. I'm in therapy and one of the things that we've been developing is the importance of relating to people, how to relate to people. I just finished reading Fosters' *Howards End*, and the epigram for that book is "only connect." It's about affections between people. That's becoming something I'm developing, but spirituality? Not so much.

Overall, I've had a great American life. It's not one that I would have traded with any other person's life. I've had adversities to overcome that other people didn't have to overcome. I faced them. I've been successful. I've been able to contribute positively to the country, not just the gay community, but to the whole country. I've been able to do things that make it easy for our community to interact with government, and to help develop our community as a model for gay communities, and I was involved in one of the biggest crises in America, which was the AIDS crisis in the '80s. I haven't done too badly for a boy from a small farm in Maryland.

I'm less satisfied with my personal relationships, my lack of a partner. That looms as something I'm really less satisfied with and that needs to be worked on. There is a quote from Jane Fonda when she went off to marry Ted Turner. She said that she's been a very successful actress, she's had all these experiences in her life, but the one experience she never had was to have a primary partnership and she wanted that in her life. That's why she gave everything to do that. I understood that; that spoke very strongly to me.

ANTHONY

"There Has to Be Something Else to This"

I WILL BE 60 IN A FEW WEEKS. I was born here in Chicago—never lived anywhere else. I completed two semesters of junior college and then I got caught up in exploring my sexuality and that over took my life. I was still able to hold on to a job. I was a mental health technician. I've been living with HIV now since 1990. If you were to ask me before protease inhibitors came along, when I was having a whole lot of health issues, if I were to make it to 2012, I would have said, "Why are you being so cruel to me? You know I'm going to die in a couple of years! Why would you even say that to me?" But I'm still here and I'm relatively healthy at this point.

One thing that is very significant in my own personal life, with my aging syndrome, is that I've articulated my faith. I've always felt a connection to Jesus; I'm a devout Christian. I was raised a Christian and my parents made me go to church. I had no spiritual connection back then. It was all intellectual. "OK, this is what people do." It wasn't until I got my diagnosis and after watching too many of my friends die, literally, in front and around me, that I said, "There has to be something else to this." I articulated my faith since then. That has been the nucleus of my survival, along with the prescription drugs that I take and my doctor's help. I have a wonderful doctor, but it has to be the grace of God that I'm still here. I have even questioned God, because I had friends who had children, who were loving parents, and God took them away. I could not understand it. I couldn't understand why God would leave me here, child free. Why would he take them? I know that you can't question God, and God's ways are not our ways, et cetera, et cetera.

I'm also a student of the scripture. I identify with the apostle Paul. Not to get on a religious vein, but in the Bible, Paul has no mission having a significant other. Maybe that's my journey, too, because I have no significant other. I haven't had one in years and I don't see it happening. But, I'll never say never.

The aging thing, interestingly enough—it's both frustrating and rewarding. I'm certainly wiser than I was even 5 years ago, let alone 15, 20 years ago, when I was in my 20s and 30s. I look at the world differently now. I feel I do have something to offer. I do let my Jesus light shine.

I had a thought on the way here to this interview. I took a bus here. There was this little kid that got on the bus. When I was about 5 or 6 years old, there was a new school being built by my home. (I'm the younger of two sons. My mother back then, in the '50s, was a housewife raising her two boys. I come from a two-parent family.) Me and my little friend Ricky—I'll never forget it—we got caught in the construction of the new school. You know, being little boys, we were over there playing. Of course, I didn't tell my mother where

I was, so she panicked and called the police. The police found us and brought us home.

I remember the policeman asking me, "Why would you not tell your mother where you were going? " In a policeman, authoritative voice he said, "You know that she was worried about you?"

I said, "Well, officer, I wasn't lost. She was the one that was lost."

I had a good childhood. However, one significant thing I do remember about my childhood was my first same-sex experience, which had to be—I think I was about 8 or 9 years old. There was another little boy in the neighborhood and we would experiment with each other's penises, just playing with them, but it felt good. He was the same age, so it wasn't a child abuse thing. I remember my older brother busting us. He humiliated me so bad. He called me every name in the book, every name but a child of God, and that sort of traumatized me for a while. He didn't tell our parents, but he told me that that's something we shouldn't be doing. Ironically, we had in the neighborhood what at that time was called a "neighborhood sissy." He was a very effeminate boy and everybody sort of tormented him.

I had both parents at home. Both of them were very loving to me, and my brother was OK until that event. He would still be a brother to me, but not as close as we were when we were both young. I never forgot that first experience. That just stuck with me.

I think I really started looking at boys sexually, I'll say, maybe seventh and eighth grade. We were still grabbing each other's boobies and crotches, but we saw that as normal. It was very pleasurable for me. Fast-forward to high school, I'm going into my second trauma with same-sex attraction. I'll never forget. I was in the locker room, after gym and we were changing. I remember fixating on this one guy who had a very blessed body. He saw me looking at him and, in front of everybody else, he humiliated me by asking me what was I looking at, but not like that, he said, "What the fuck are you looking at? You motherfucker!" I just sort of backed my way out of the locker room. Thank goodness he didn't want to get physical. He just got loud and, of course, all the boys were laughing. That was my second little trauma—first year in high school.

Then I decided I was crazy. I decided this is not right; I shouldn't be having these thoughts. I tried to repress them, started smoking cigarettes, gained weight, and there was absolutely no one I could talk to about it. We didn't have any of the services we have nowadays, even though it still could be better, but it certainly was not like that in the '60s.

I was also into girls, but I was a good actor back then. I had girlfriends. I know it's hard to believe this middle-age shell you see now, but I used to be good looking, back in the day before I had these dimples from the side effects of HIV treatment. I used to be a good looking guy. I always had wonderful female relationships.

I've only had two female sexual experiences and they were both way out of high school. The first one I was about 21 and the second one was once the epidemic really started, when it went from gay cancer to AIDS. That scared me and led me to think that maybe I need to retrace my orientation. I made a feeble attempt. I thought to myself that the best way to do it was to try and find a bisexual woman, and I did. We talked about it and we had one sexual encounter, and afterward we both sort of agreed that it was mediocre for both of us. Actually, that was my first and only experience with cunnilingus. The first sexual experience I had with a female was strictly missionary. That was kind of funny, looking back on it now. We both agreed that it was just OK, nothing spectacular; no fireworks went off. I've always been able to communicate with women and I find it amazing that sometimes gay men say, "Ugh! You had sex with a woman?" That's such a turnoff to them. It didn't work for me, but I still tried it.

One significant thing that did happen in high school that really brought me to my orientation was in my junior year. I met a senior who introduced me to adult same-sex relations. I was just a toy to him, looking back at it. What I mean by that is that he pursued me; he knew he was my first. I was so excited that I ejaculated too soon, just by the time we got our clothes off. The good part about being a teenager is that all I needed was 2 minutes to be ready again. After a couple or three times, he lost interest. I was no longer a challenge to him. I allowed him to overwhelm me. That was a trauma. I didn't handle that well. "What did I do?"

I went to the neighborhood effeminate guy, who always had a little crave for me anyway. I told him that I had these feelings and he said, "Oh yes, you're gay. You need to come to this party with me." And he took me to my first party. "Oh, you're going to be fine. You just need to go to this gay party."

It was a house party; it wasn't at a bar. I'm, like, 16 maybe and the guys were 20 and up. He left me at the party. Here I'm this little lamb among these wolves! I'm 16 years old, nice, tender, and good looking. And these older guys, of course they're going to—and that's what happened. One did push up on me and took me home. Had sex with me and made me feel real good, but at that time I also had a girlfriend. He told me to stay in the closet. He encouraged me to keep the girlfriend, but he also told me that he had a boyfriend. This was just a one-night thing. So I'm thinking, "What is this gay stuff?"

My friend, the effeminate guy, and I started hanging out. He was into promiscuous anonymous sex and I jumped on that bandwagon. Oh man, he introduced me to Grant Park cruising, bathhouses, and I just went cuckoo crazy. It's a miracle I'm here. I started going out to bars and I'd get home at about maybe 5 or 6 o'clock in the morning, when as soon as you hit the pillow you go into that REM sleep.

Well, my father let me sleep for about maybe 20 minutes and then he'd wake me up, "Where have you been?" (And you never talked back to my father.) "Were you out with your faggot friends?"

I said "Yeah, what about it?"

My mother was crying. She was hysterical. And we never discussed it, after I calmed my mother down. It was never discussed that, yes, I am this way and all of that. They just sort of put it on the back burner and I, of course, never brought it up.

Then my brother and I had another confrontation. I was on the phone once and I called my friend "honey." He gave me a slap in the face. I've worn glasses since I was 12, and my glasses flew off my face and hit the basement door. I've always been afraid of my brother, too. I just packed my little stuff, and I had a couple of friends that had a wonderful, huge apartment in the south of Chicago, and they let me stay there for a few days until things cooled down.

My mother begged me to come back home, so I did. We had a discussion, "This is how I am." They all thought I was going through a phase. They sort of accepted it in the way that they knew how, which is "OK, we hear you." It was

"Don't ask; don't discuss." "You said this now; don't ever bring it up." "Don't throw it out in front of the other family and friends." "Keep that on the DL." I got that message quite right. I moved out when I was 19 for sure. I have not lived with my parents since.

However, sometime in my 30s—. I had never told my father that I loved him. I know he knew that, and I know he loved me, and I don't recall him telling me that he loved me. I went through an epiphany in my 30s. "You need to do this." And I did. I asked him to come to my place by himself, and I said to him, "I know that you don't care for my lifestyle, but I also feel that you still love me. It would be nice to hear it sometimes. I just want to let you know that I love you and I don't think I've ever told you that blah, blah, blah." I felt that that was a milestone for the both of us.

I worked for a major airline from 1979 to 1994—wonderful job, wonderful benefits. I loved the experience; however, I was in a different head back then and I had one particular supervisor who was excellent at pushing my buttons. I did not give him the respect he deserved as a supervisor. That's my biggest regret today. I got fired or, as they tell me now at headquarters when I call about my pension, "you separated." So we became separated in 1994; they divorced me. That's my biggest regret.

I'm not dark skinned; I'm a nice mocha, a nice coffee—not that there's anything wrong with dark skin. I love my dark-skinned brothers and sisters. One incident that I remember is trying to get into a gay bar on Broadway—this was the '70s—and they had a card issue, but it seemed that they carded African Americans more so than any other group.

The disheartening thing was that the guy at the door, who was carding mostly black people and rejecting mostly black people, was black himself. That was beyond trauma, because here is somebody your own kind, "No you can't come in here 'cause you're black." White people behind me were getting in—they obviously were much younger—without showing ID. You always see skin color before you see orientation. Other times you can mask your orientation; you can't deny that you are black or African American.

The larger society is so youth oriented anyway, and what also makes me not go to bars any more is that now, at my age, men my age, who I might be attracted to, are looking for the younger guys. They'd tell me, "Oh, you're too old, babe." It's discouraging and disheartening. And of course, nowadays there is so much online stuff you can do. I'm only on one site. I'm familiar with the sex hookup sites and, trust me, sex is very, very important still to me. But, because I'm positive, I have had a couple of men tell me they couldn't handle that. They told me they were negative and they definitely had to have someone who also was negative. I can respect that, but it still hurts. But I'll get over it.

In the site that I'm on now, you post personal ads. Well, unfortunately, I've noticed that the people I flirt with—you know, someone who is age appropriate, unless I read the profile and it says age is not an issue—are not interested in me. It's always something. I'm ever hopeful.

My facial lipodystrophy is an issue for me. Everybody else says, "Oh it's not that bad." But I look at my face all the time and I see it all the time. When I smile you see the wrinkles, and I'm going to be 60 in a couple of weeks. To me, I look like I'm 70. But, I have learned, through prayer and meditation: "You know, you can't afford the procedure to fix it, so get over it. Be grateful you're still here. It could be worse." That's how I try to live my life. That's how I handle this aging thing. It's not easy for me, because I haven't had a significant other since—I can't remember his name—that's awful! It's been at least 10 years. Now, of course, I have little sex buddies and I hook up sometimes, but I want my man.

Back in the '80s, I was in a relationship. Looking back on that relationship it was not—even though we were probably under the illusion that it was romance involved, it was basically just a sexual relationship. Back then, I was sort of apathetic about HIV because it was mostly white males who were dying. You didn't hear of too many black people dying until I had a friend who happened to be into white men and he got the virus. He went straight down. Then, of course, every day you heard about more and more cases. So we didn't change our behavior and I was not true to him. I know, I had a promiscuous, nonmonogamous type of attitude about sex. I don't know if he was aware of that then, and I'm not sure he was monogamous. We didn't come together and say "Hey, we need to make some changes." Again, very few black people that we knew—and this is a stereotype—but we always thought it would be the white boys who got sick, until it started hitting home, closer and closer, until our friends started getting it. Again, that did not change our behavior.

Don't ask; don't tell. It's not right at our doorstep, so why bring it up? Why give it energy? Actually, I never stopped having promiscuous anonymous sex. I just kept going. Sometime in 1990, my late best friend, who was bisexual, became infected and he could not handle AZT (azidothymidine, a type of antiretroviral drug). Needless to say, the disease just took him right over. I was in shock and denial at the same time.

I wish we could find a cure. To be honest, at this point, I've joined support groups. I've done all kinds of experimental things. I feel like I'm overloaded with HIV and AIDS information. I have no interest at all in working directly with HIV/AIDS organizations. I'm just overloaded. I'm tired of hearing about how so-and-so has got the virus now or so-and-so died last weekend. I'm tired of hearing stories. I'm not cynical and I'm not hard-hearted, but I just can't see me doing another support group.

I have an older, heterosexual female friend who I used to work with. She is retired now, but she's got lots of health issues. She's 16 years my senior, so she's old enough to be my mother. We call each other like sister and brother; she's never had a brother and I've never had any sisters. We've known each other over 25 years now; we are very close. Needless to say, she knows all about my orientation and, interestingly, I just found out that—I've known this woman for over 25 years, she's always known me as the same-gender, gay-loving man—she, up until a couple of years ago, thought I wanted to be a woman. She thought all gay men wanted to be women. I had to educate her.

I do get in the basement sometimes with my depression. I don't have anybody. There is no romantic significant other, and that's what I long for. That is my heart's desire. In fact, I don't think I would feel comfortable talking to my female friend about that. My friend in New York is in a different mind-set because he is negative. I feel that negative people don't really understand. I have an ex-boyfriend who is in California now and he's positive. He is 10 years my senior.

On some things, I could talk to him about. I met him at an HIV spiritual retreat, back in 1999, and we just connected. But, we got caught up in that initial romantic thing and then we grew apart. But even now, we are not as close as we used to be 2 years ago. We were together for 9 months and he has a new boyfriend now; he's had several boyfriends since he and I broke up. He's done the heterosexual thing in terms of marriage. He has grown children and grandchildren. There are times when I wish I could call him and I say, "Hey, this is going on. Can you help me out?" I never get so depressed that I can't function. I have my faith. I always know that this, too, shall pass. I always have to keep moving.

I've been positive since 1990 and I've had this damn diabetes. I hate diabetes! I have a much harder time with that than with HIV. By the grace of God I'm undetectable and I have been for years. I love food, and food is such a comfort. I like healthy food, I like greasy food, I like sugary food, I like sugar-free food, but again, everything is turned into—I hate diabetes! I hate it more than HIV. I'm slowly getting that under control, too, because my glucose is a little up there. I'm very grateful for the health I have.

The most I'm satisfied with is that I have articulated my faith. I know Jesus loves me as a same-gender loving man. I've been beat up like so many of us with religion. "You're going to hell because you like men." I know in my spirit that's not true. The greatest thing that I think I've accomplished, in my almost 60 years on this Earth, is that I know what my purpose is: to love God first, with all my being, and, in a like manner, love you and all other human beings. I love God unconditionally.

MARVIN

"I Learned Very Early That It's Not Just about Being Gay"

I DO ANYTHING I CAN possibly do for living. I am under the sum of the Great Recession. I lost a job last November. I was asked by a cousin to come to work with him selling credit card processing equipment and I am not being successful with it. A lot of my time is spent doing odd jobs, like painting houses. After the recent flood in Chicago, I cleaned up a basement to earn money. I needed cash immediately because my savings have run out. I'm on unemployment, but those payments are just $157 every 2 weeks. My mortgage is behind and my house is in foreclosure. Luckily, I own my car free and clear.

This is a terrible situation and it's the first time in my life that I've been in this condition. It has lasted throughout every month of 2010. Up until the end of 2009, I could live on savings. But now, a new company has come to Chicago, and I signed up to work with them in June, after going and working at the Census Bureau for 6 weeks. I have made two sales with them so far in August, but I anticipate being able to make more sales. The problem is that I do not own a laptop;

I own a desktop computer. I desperately need a laptop computer with wireless Internet so I can make sales outside my home. Literally, I have like $30 in the bank and $100 in my pocket, and that's it. Those $100 dollars need to build up so that on the 17th of August I can pay the mortgage, which I negotiated down by 50%—so, $822. I can't afford a laptop. I have to save money to make the mortgage on the 17th or else. I will lose my house in a court hearing on the 23rd of August.

It is the Great Depression Part II, brought about by multimillionaire bankers who want a person like me to let them make a million dollars a year, plus a $7000 bonus every year at Christmastime. Life is hell, in terms of finances.

I have promised to all my friends to hang in there and hope that something happens. But I'm desperate at this moment. It's like society wants your last dime. And so, financially, I make money by doing odd jobs and selling wireless 4G computers, modems, cell phones, but I can't even afford $300 to buy the equipment that I'm selling. I hope that I have enough friends who will buy from me, so that at least I can buy the product, too, and get a laptop. This American capitalist system is the worst system devised, letting people fall off the wagon completely. There is no help out there to speak of.

From 1991 until 2003, I was a store manager. Things were going great until December 2005. All store managers were called up to a hotel. We were given this fantastic steak-and-potatoes dinner, which we came to call the Last Supper, because the CEO got up and said: "Effective tomorrow, all 32 stores in Chicago are closed." Come 2006, I got in a temporary agency and worked various jobs: under a 90-day contract I'd do telemarketing, then another 90-day contract would come along and I'd do something else. So that worked for a while. I went from being employed by a mattress giant to working as a car salesman. In 2008 the stock market crashed; loans froze up. The banks required customers, in early 2008, to have a credit score of 620 to get financing on a new Mustang. In summer 2008, they required a 720 credit score. I could not make sales and my other salespeople had a lot of customers who wanted to buy but couldn't get financed. After this kept happening month after month, the dealer closed and we all lost our jobs.

So I said, "OK. What can I do now?" Monster.com, Carreerbuilder.com, and, sure enough, I got a call from a cemetery. I literally was selling cemetery plots, niches, and mausoleums where cremation ashes can be stored indefinitely. Yet, very few people were willing to pay $100, even $50 per month on a burial plot. That was not high on their priority list, so I couldn't make enough sales to get traction there. I started living off savings and that's how I got to this point.

I'm 56 years old. I was born in North Carolina. I lived there until I was in junior high school. Then, we moved out of the state, where I completed high school. I went to a state university and finished my BA in '76 at a great school. Those were the four most fantastic years of my life; I loved it. I've lived in Chicago since 1996.

The good thing is that, as you age, you get wisdom that comes from living, experiencing, and understanding. I can be philosophical about things that are going on in the world—and I'm not a person who loves to do anything more than to read; I love to read. That is the number one thing about aging, that you are moving further and further into this future that we all dreamed about and now is here.

Unfortunately, the thing that comes to my mind is that I am a man who is attracted to other men. I came out of the closet when I was 18 years old, at college, and I've been out ever since. That means that when I came out, no one had yet heard of AIDS or HIV, but I experienced it starting in the summer of 1981. I was a very outgoing person, gave lots of dinner parties at my home, went out to social events, liked to party, liked to dance, liked to enjoy life, met all kinds of people, and enjoyed the freedom that living in a big city brings. But from 1981 until 2010, 158 people that I knew personally died of HIV-related causes. And I know that number so well because I have kept a list in a Bible that my mother gave me when I graduated from college. She said that, throughout life, if there's anything that you can't control, just give it to the Lord. I could not control all these deaths. They were devastating. There were 158 of them. I know when each person died or was celebrated. I remember their names, I remember their personalities, and I remember the good times with them.

But, that is the thing about aging that is bad. As an HIV-negative person, I have outlived so many people by years now—people who died when they and I were in our 30s, 40s, and early 50s. They're gone. I had always expected that by making a lot of good friends, I'd have a lot of friends my age in my 60s, 70s, and 80s. Some people in our family have lived into their 80s and I have one great-great-grandfather who lived to be 106. But lately, diabetes has come into my life and I understand now, after the fact, that exactly from the year 1827 until the year 1933, when my great-great-grandfather was living, people had no fast foods and no instant sugary Coca-Cola and Pepsi. People ate basic fruits and vegetables. He had a healthy diet, and that's changed, in a fast age when you want to pick up a bite on the go; there were no drive-ins then.

In June 1981, my cousin, who had been distancing himself from me when I came out (he was rather homophobic), sent me a newspaper clipping from the *Detroit Free Press*: "Rare Cancer Strikes Gay Men." He said, "I hope you don't get this because it sounds really bad." I read the article and it was describing what they called the HTLV (human T-lymphotropic virus III) back then. In 1983 I actually met someone who disclosed to me that he was living with HIV, and so it became more personal.

I read that unprotected anal sex was a leading contributor to HIV transmission. And it made sense. So I said, "Well, I am terrified of AIDS, I am scared of getting HIV, so perhaps if I get involved in a lover relationship and both of us are tested negative, I simply will not trust a condom. If HIV is going to cause me to go through this horrible death that I am seeing, I will not trust a condom. I will just not have anal sex. Period."

One of my nicest childhood memories is one that's actually preserved in pictures that I found in my mother's house when she died. The picture was about the day my mother bought her first brand-new car. It was a 1957 Plymouth Savoy, and the picture shows me. I was sitting on the back of this car and my arm was wrapped around this tail fin.

My father married three times. My mother was his second wife. Why did he marry and divorce, and marry and divorce?

Because he was a violent man. He committed assault and battery against my mother and she left him while still pregnant with me. She moved out. My grandparents were of retirement age. My grandmother was a teacher and my grandfather was principal of a school. At that time, in the 1950s, a teaching job provided a solid middle-class income, so I grew up in a solid middle-class home.

My mother feared that African American high schools would be closed when they were desegregated, and that's exactly what happened in many cities in the South. In 1964, '65, and '66, the African American high schools were turned into grade schools, and all the high school students went to the previously all-white schools. Unfortunately, many of the African American teachers were not hired to work in the all-white schools. So, my mother actively looked for employment, and that's why we moved to another state. We again lived a very comfortable middle-class life. My grandparents stayed in North Carolina.

In college, I worked to earn one third of my tuition. I got a scholarship that paid one third of the tuition and the other one third my mother gave me from her savings. In college I was doing well, and throughout my life in Chicago from 1976 all the way up to 2008, I was doing well.

I had lots and lots of friends. I used to play Little League Baseball; I was in the Cub Scouts. Every Sunday I was required to go to Sunday school for children, from the time I was in first grade all the way through my teenage years. Then, in the summertime, the Baptist church had what they called summer vacation bible school, and we went to school 5 days a week from morning until afternoon. I met a lot of children doing that. It was fun; it was good. In high school

I was on the basketball team, in the Spanish club, on the student council, and in the political science club. I was just very involved. I had lots and lots of friends all the time.

I had a Western Flyer bicycle and so I was able to go all over town. It was a small town. Back in the 1950s and '60s, streets were safe; parents didn't worry about Amber Alerts and all that. I loved to move around and see things and do things, and I had a bicycle, so I could get around. Then, I was always taller than everybody else in my class; I was expected to play basketball, football, and track. And I did. I enjoyed sports.

The main focus of religion at that time was: It's very important to live in a way that you would be respected, never tell a lie, never steal anything, and never mistreat other people. Those were the things that we were taught very, very thoroughly—and that the most shameful thing in the world was to go to jail. You never wanted to do anything that could possibly cause you to go to jail. That also was a fear of the white-dominated prison system in the South. That was what religion meant to me.

I realized when I was 13, in an instant, that I was gay. One day, my two friends and I were at a convenience store, and off on the side there was a magazine rack and they were looking at *Playboy*, showing seminude women, and I wasn't paying attention to the magazines. But, I had found a magazine with body builders who were all men. They noticed and they said, "Why are you looking at that?" I was busted!

From that point on, it became a constant awareness. I had to avoid any kind of problems by making sure that people wouldn't notice if I wasn't showing some interest in women. And actually it caused no problems in my family because I learned very quickly what locker room jokes were about. I knew when to laugh and when not to laugh. I could understand the whole thing because I felt a little outside of everybody else's world. It made me see and understand what I needed to do to maintain my popularity.

At the same time, I will never forget that one Sunday in 1969, on the front page of the local newspaper there was a picture, with people at a distance, showing the Stonewall riots: "Homosexuals Riot Against Police in New York City." There was no article, just a headline, but I said, "Those people are like me." I said, "Alright, I need to move to a big city so I can meet people like that." So, my number one thought in mind all the time when I was a teenager: "I have to finish high school; I have to move to a big city. If possible, I have to go to college so I can be free to move around and not get stuck in this place."

When I was in high school, there was one guy in my class who was noticeably effeminate and people would tell locker room jokes about him. I was afraid to make him my friend. I didn't want people to think that I was gay and interested in an effeminate man. Then there was another guy in our school who was very interested in the Wallace-for-president campaign in 1968. Wallace was, at the time, the governor of Alabama and he wanted to abolish the civil rights laws at the federal level; he was totally against racial integration. So I knew at that moment that I needed to leave that city because there were a lot of people who didn't even want me to be in the school because I'm black. I learned very early that it's not just about being gay; there are these bigger issues.

In the South, I clearly remember seeing stores that said "whites only," and you just could not go into the store.

I remembered traveling by bus and everyone black had to sit in the colored waiting room. There were separate rooms for black passengers in buses and trains. At the movie theater you could not sit on the first floor; all the black people had to sit in the balcony. You could not go buy popcorn at the counter. You would have to go down the stairs and knock on a door that was behind the popcorn counter. I vividly remember being treated very differently during segregation.

When I went to Chicago, I started attending the Good Shepherd Parish Metropolitan Community Church. I went there every Sunday because, throughout my life, I'd been taught that it's important to go to church on Sunday and acknowledge the gifts that you've gotten from God. I met a lot of people. I joined the Illinois Gay and Lesbian Rights Task Force and met a lot of people there. I went to a gay rights rally in Washington, DC, in 1979. I remember going to the 1987 march in Washington to see the AIDS quilt. And I went to the 1993 march on Washington.

I've never had a partner. It never occurred to me to live with someone, until I met an individual I started to date. He moved in, but we never got to the point of forming a relationship because he is one of the people who developed HIV. In 1988 he moved out; he died in 1991.

I had another boyfriend, who lived right down the street. We were very, very close. We had a long-lasting gay relationship, but we never moved in together. Once again, in 1993, he didn't answer his phone. I called yet again and again, later to find out that he was in the hospital. He died in March 1993.

So those were two potential relationships that ended before they got a chance to develop. Over the years, that has happened again and again—potential relationships—but before they develop, my potential partner dies. That's why I focus on those 158 people on my list—so many possible relationships, but it just didn't happen.

I always have been a positive, optimistic person. I think I developed that way of thinking through going to church each week. If you pray, if you strive to do your best, if you always help people and meet people, things will turn out OK, and that has been a very effective way of living. Things have turned out well. I have gotten employment when I needed it, because I knew someone and they knew someone. Currently, what is keeping me motivated to live from day to day is the thought that I did not cause the stock market crash; I did not bundle derivatives and sell them off because the Glass–Steagall Act got repealed. These are things that happened way beyond my scope of influence. So I should not feel responsible for the economic situation. I think it's time for the multibillion-dollar Wall Street bankers to be held accountable, and that's how I'm going to approach life. Life has gotten tough; I need to get tougher.

Illinois was the first state in 1961 to repeal the sodomy law that made consenting sex between same-sex partners not criminal. That was a part of the reason why I moved to Chicago. Once in Chicago, I learned about the Society for Human Rights, which was formed back in the 1920s—the first gay rights group in the country. I got involved and volunteered with them. I went to Springfield and spoke about discrimination. The story I told was that, in 1978, I went to a TV show and talked about a new group called the National Coalition of Black Gays. The next day, Monday morning, someone had told my boss that I was on this talk show and that I was gay. I was put on probation and, at the end of the 90-day probation, I was let go. I went to Springfield, to the Chicago City Council, and other places to talk about the fact that it's wrong that when someone exercises the freedom of speech, there are economic consequences because of discrimination.

As time went by, the National Coalition of Black Gays kind of faded away, but in 1986, a group of black men in Philadelphia formed a group called *Adodi.* In the Yoruba language of Nigeria, it means two-spirited man. It was formed because Reagan was in the White House and did not say anything about HIV. *Adodi* said we need to do something on our own to address AIDS among black men in Philadelphia. I found out about the *Adodi* retreats in the early '90s. It was a group of people who, yes, they were working on HIV issues, but also were networking as writers, actors, singers, and people in the arts. I kept going to *Adodi* retreats year after year after year to this date.

At the Center on Halsted [the community center for LGBT people in Chicago], I saw a little card offering counseling services at Howard Brown [the Howard Brown Health Center for LGBT people in Chicago]. I've gone once a week for the past 2 years. I told the counselor that I want to live into the future; I want to live again; however, I will not leave my house. I told her that if the day comes when this foreclosure proceeding gets to the point where I'm evicted from my house that I paid for, for 11 years, I would buy a gun and I would have one shot to the heart. That is my motivation to negotiate with the mortgage company. I'm not going to move. I will not move. I will live in that house until the day I die and, if they put me out, that's the day I die.

In 2007, I lost my health insurance. My diabetes spiked all the way to a blood glucose level of 310. I had stopped buying and taking Metformin (to treat type 2 diabetes). Right now I buy a generic Metformin—just $4 a month—and I got a doctor at County Hospital to prescribe it.

What I really need is a dentist. I've lost teeth because of the diabetes and not being able to take the medicine for about a year or so. A dentist said I should get all the teeth pulled and get dentures. Yeah, but that's $5000 that I don't have. Always keep aspirin in the house for pain.

Last year I self-published a book on same-gender loving black men. The book tells the story of how same-gender loving people provide power within the African American community. I want to write a sequel to that book. I need to do it based on the feedback I got from my first book. That's my goal in life: to write my next book. I will channel my anger into writing a book.

I have my health. I woke up this morning able to walk, to talk, to live. The meds have kept the diabetes under control. I own my car, so I can travel and go wherever I want to. I went to Michigan in my car this past year to the *Adodi* retreat. As I said, *Adodi* has been a sustaining group in my life. I go to a lesbian- and gay-affirming Baptist church. I'm happy that I am in my house at this moment, and my house is that close to my heart. I'm happy that on the 4th of July weekend 30 people came over, and we cooked hot dogs and hamburgers on a grill in my backyard. It's very important to me that when I throw a party, lots of people come over and they have a good time. Two weeks ago, another friend invited me to his party. I'm so happy that I have friends that invite me to parties and dinners and to have a very good time. Life is great, except for the mortgage and the issues surrounding it.

ROBERT

"I'm a Pusher and I Don't Like to Hear the Word No"

I'M 65 AND HAD 12 YEARS OF CATHOLIC SCHOOL, then 4 years of secular college at a university. I look back on that and I can't figure out why I was so enamored with the religion, unless it was just the routine and the ceremony and being surrounded by it all day at school. As soon as I graduated from high school, that was the end of formal religion for me. Right now I believe in God and I will talk versus pray. It's just not important right now.

I financed my way through college by being a hair dresser. I got my BA and found out that I was able to make more money continuing as a hair dresser. So that's exactly what I did do, and I wound up working for a large beauty company. Now I'm retired and work part time for an LGBT social services agency with seniors.

When people say "older age," I hear "a decline in health, isolation, a decline in looks and in your physical appearance." You are being reminded that you are aging every time you look in the mirror.

Probably close with the isolationism is loss of friends. I find it more difficult to make friends as I get older because either you don't have the time to build that solid friendship that you did when you were in your 20s or 30s, or it just seems that it's harder to connect with people who, perhaps, have like experiences. Since you are not going to be at a certain age starting to build experiences together, you have to find people who have some of the same experiences so that you can relate to them easily. I think as you age that gets somewhat difficult.

My most salient memories in my childhood began with the fact that I was born with a severe cleft foot and had to go through a number of major surgeries in order to be able to walk. The entire foot had to be rebuilt from portions of my hip and bones and stuff. I was pulled to school in a wagon for kindergarten. Prior to that, I spent most of the time in hospitals or in braces. The last surgery I had was when I was 13. It really did leave a—. It actually wasn't a bad time, but it was different, I think, than other childhoods. I was homebound or in care, so I found myself around my mother and my grandmother quite a bit.

As a result of having that type of physical impairment, if you will, I chose to ignore a lot of doctor's warnings. I went into a profession of hair dressing, which required standing on my feet. To this day, I push myself because one of the prognoses that I was given was that I would probably wind up in a wheelchair when I reached my 60s because of the muscle atrophy and just the joints giving up. And I'm 65 today and I'm still maneuvering. Some of that is pushing myself. That whole period of time was very formative, because it molded my personality. I'm a pusher and I don't like to hear the word *no*. I feel that people can do what they need to do if they put their mind to it.

Actually, my family life was pretty good. I would say it was normal. Perhaps to an outsider, not so normal, because my father was younger than my mother, about 5 years, which at that time, back in 1940s, seemed larger than it is now. They were nontraditional in that my mother worked and my father did, too. Looking back, they were very colorful people. They loved to go out; we lived in the city. I had knowledge of gay people from early on. Some family members were in show business, minor league show business. It was a very comfortable sort of life.

My mother worked in retail, and then when a hospital opened here in Chicago, she became a secretary. Later on, before she retired, she was instrumental in putting together an AIDS ward for this hospital. Because of my being gay and her knowing all of my friends, she was aware. She was seeing men come into the hospital. At that time, they were dying quickly; they were developing sarcoma. She pushed an acceptance of a ward or an area. She was the first to go in and minister to these men.

My father, unfortunately, passed away at a very early age, when he was 51. I had a father up until I was in my early 20s, and then basically it was my mother and I. I was out on my own, but she also was a widow; she never remarried.

I have a brother who is younger, but—and it has nothing to do with the gay factor—we are just two distinctly different people. I think part of it had to do with the age gap between us. There were no shared experiences. We just have different lifestyles. I see him about once a month, or whatever, and we talk on the telephone maybe weekly, even if it's just a check-in call.

When I was growing up, we always lived in areas that were not close to the schools I went to, so the friends I had were few and far between. I did have one good friend as a child. He lived at the other end of the block, but I spent a great deal of my time by myself, and continue to do so today. Part of it may have been my medical condition. I had a collection of toy soldiers that I played with and Lincoln Logs, and I drew and I took art lessons. I didn't have a bunch of kids to go around with. Eventually, I learned to ride a bicycle and that gave me the biggest sense of freedom, because then I was able to go out of the block that I lived on, but I did most of that stuff by myself.

High school wasn't that bad. I had friends in high school. I suppose I would have been considered sort of popular, or whatever. I think I had to work at it a little bit to have the friends that I had. I wasn't sure if I was gay or not at the time, but I dated. I dated females—never really had a problem getting dates. I didn't really enjoy them. After high school, I dropped those friends from high school and had one good friend. I came out to him and let him know that I was gay and that ended that friendship. I sort of moved away. I don't have any—even though it wasn't a bad period of time, I have no compunction to attend a 50-year high school reunion or to see what those people are like or know about them. My life took off in an entirely different direction. That's when I think my life really started to begin as it is today. Where some people still have close ties with maybe high school or college folks, I don't.

As I said, I came out to my best friend because we were out of school then. We were both finishing college and I realized that I was attracted to men and he was definitely heterosexual. I just felt that being as close friends as we were, this is something that I could share with him, that he would understand and we could move forward as friends. One evening, I approached the subject with him and told him that I was gay. "I'm thinking of dating men, seeing men in a sexual manner." He became very upset and asked me to leave, and I did. That was the last communication I had with him.

If I look back, I probably was attracted to men as a child. I loved to play with toy soldiers, cowboys, and Indians. I had a whole set of cowboys and Indians. Back in the day, there were these big biblical epics and movies, like *Samson and Delilah*, and I was fascinated with watching the gladiators and the men in the robes. The storyline could be very thin, but I was just wondering what was underneath those robes. When I look back on it, it's probably a very early time that I realized that maybe there was something there.

When I really decided to act on my instincts, there were some issues. I had been seeing a psychologist (this was after my father passed away). We talked about my sexuality and I had broached the subject to him that I thought that I was a gay male. He said, "Well, we can fix that." He got down a medical book and explained to me about a woman's clitoris—where to find it and how wonderful this was all going to be. I actually was really appalled; it really upset me. This was part of someone's anatomy I wanted to know nothing about. It just absolutely turned me off. When I left there I thought, "You know what? He did me a service, in that I was convinced now that I was on the right track and there was no going the other way." Again, my parents were very understanding, so I didn't have a problem there. The transition, if there is a transition from straight to gay life, was fairly comfortable.

I was fortunate in having a career as a hair dresser at a particular time when being gay, being a male, and being a hair dresser was a status thing. It was considered very fashionable. You were accepted. You moved into areas that maybe would not be open to other people.

My initial venture into gay life was to a drop-in center. At that time, it was located in Old Town in Chicago, and I went there to a couple of drop-in meetings and decided that this wasn't really the type of people I wanted to associate with. I started going to bars. I met a number of gentlemen who were somewhat older than me. I was probably early 20s and let's say they were 30, or whatever. The attraction on their part may have been sexual, but we later became friends. Some of them I still see to this day. There was a mentoring process that took place. It was through them that I learned my way around the gay world: the bars, the bathhouses, restaurants to go to, how to eat, how to dress, where to shop. It really was like having a teacher.

There was a very big bar scene. There were discos and actually elaborate bars. We were out almost all the time. I belonged to a very social set of people that were out. Then, being in the hair-dressing business, it became apparent that people were getting sick. A friend of ours came down with AIDS, but we all thought it was cancer. He got very ill very quickly. We still partied on, but he was fading fast. That's when we started realizing this could be this AIDS epidemic that people were talking about, and one in our group had gotten it. He passed away rather quickly. His parents came from out of town and took his body away. They wouldn't allow a burial or a service where he lived. In fact, they wouldn't acknowledge that their son had died of this new disease.

From there, I just watched other friends and acquaintances acquire the disease and, little by little, pass away. I lost a great number of friends during that period of time.

My feelings at that time, naturally, were of sorrow and of loss. I can't tell you how many chapels I sat in and cried, or chapels that I sat there and laughed because some of the ceremonies were right off the wall. I mean, with a disco ball and the whole thing.

I often wondered, "Why them not me?" There wasn't much difference in the sexual behaviors and the drinking. I didn't know about a lot of drugs, but the behaviors were similar. I seemed to float above it all. To this day, I kind of wonder why I escaped without any sort of illness. "Why did I escape HIV/AIDS?"

I have to go back to a master plan set in motion by someone other than myself. Later in life, I took care of my mother. I was her primary caregiver for quite a number of years. Maybe that was part of the plan. And maybe part of the plan was for me to live to old age and relate this story; I don't know. I don't know, but my life didn't end then and I don't see it ending soon now.

HIV is a managed disease. I think research and medical therapies help overcome a lot of the symptoms. Today, I don't think it can be cured, but I think it's maybe a chronic situation that people now can live with, instead of this sudden death sentence that was apparent at the beginning of the epidemic. I don't relate to HIV/AIDS that much at this age, because I'm not that sexual anymore. It seems that I am past that phase in my life. I may be kidding myself. I'm not sure. I'm glad I wasn't part of it. I feel relieved that I escaped the disease.

When I started with the beauty company was a big step. I went from being really a party person, a club person, to having a career. I remember various promotions I got along the way. It began to shape me in a much different way. And there was a lover of mine at the time that pushed me in that direction. He was a successful man. I think that influences, today, who I am and my values. If that hadn't happened, I probably would have stayed in the club scene and, eventually, I think, would have drifted into more promiscuous relationships and perhaps wound up with HIV.

Within my company, I felt comfortable enough and had enough status that I got the company involved in the first AIDS Walk in Chicago. There were like 12 or 13 of us with a banner from the company. That grew to where upward of 100 people marched in years to come, and the company contributed a lot of money.

I bought a building with my partner. We broke up. I had a vacant apartment in the building and my mother had sold her home, so she moved into the apartment. It was going to be a transitional thing. She liked the arrangement; I liked the arrangement. She stayed on for 20 years. At the end, the last number of years she was ill.

What's helped me get through life and go over the obstacles is a personal sense of "I can do it." I have to do it, because I am only me. There is no partner. There is no family. The friendship connection has dwindled, so it's very important that I rely on myself and my own resources to overcome whatever obstacles I've faced and what obstacles I foresee in the future. Some of it is economics and some of it includes coping mechanisms. I deal with almost daily pain in my legs. You just learn to have a mantra or something like that to help you overcome it. I don't feel good unless I push myself. I am not a sympathetic person as a result of that—not at all. That sort of drive is what keeps me going. Had I realized this when I was younger, in my 20s and 30s and making money and spending it freely in the clubs, I would have worked harder and been more focused. How much better off I would be today! But I did OK.

My general health is fine. I've just been diagnosed with rheumatoid arthritis, and that bothers me because it's a difficult disease to cure. I don't believe there is a cure; you can go through certain remissions. I shy away from the medication because medications break down your immune system and, as a result, I don't take them. I fear loss of mobility due to that disease, where I have to be wheelchair bound or something like that.

I'm going to reinvent myself. I have plans. I have a plan to look into some cosmetic surgery. I'm thinking of relocating, just going on to another chapter in my life. Definitely, I'm moving to a better weather place, and just the fact that I need to keep active. The winters here in Chicago are so long they limit your ability to be active. I may relocate or look into spending a certain amount of time in a better climate in the winter.

I don't know whether I will meet another partner and I'm not sure I want to take on the responsibility or am ready to compromise anymore in my life. It would be great to enlarge my circle of friends. I'm still sexually active with anonymous partners. So, that part I have a release for. Right now I feel very selfish about the life that I have. Having another partner doesn't play into it.

As I age, the LGBT issue, for me personally, my sexual orientation, is not that important. It seems to be lessening. I find that as I age and I meet people who are straight, the sexual orientation doesn't seem to be as important as maybe the economic factor, the personality factor, the history. There's a little bit of a stumbling block when it comes to family and grandchildren. But I found that—for example, I live in a building and it's a small kind of building, and everybody knows that I'm gay, and as long as I can afford to live there, and I look like everybody there, I fit in. It doesn't matter to anybody. When I travel, I find the same thing. I have gay friends, we go out to gay places, but the exclusivity doesn't need to be there anymore. I feel as comfortable in a straight bar as in a gay bar. I don't know that I could ever be a flag waver anymore, oddly enough.

The greatest satisfaction in my life is that I'm financially secure. I took care of my mother and did not have to place her in a nursing home, which was her wish and mine. I like where I live and I'm looking forward to the next, I believe, 20 years or so.

And this is so vain. I've gained so much weight. Nobody would recognize me if I show them old pictures. This just came up when I turned 60. I'm over 6 feet and weighed 165 lb. Model thin! And I had jet-black hair. That is disconcerting to me, because I feel I am that person, but I don't look like that person. It's hard for me to put the two together.

That's why I'm considering some plastic surgery and re-invention. I want to get a little closer to who that person was. Otherwise, I'm fairly content. I am lonely at times, but I realize that loneliness is the price I pay for my personal freedom.

RAMIRO

"My Family Is Really My Gay Friends"

I'M 56 YEARS OLD AND I WAS born in Chicago. My father is from Mexico; he came here during the '40s. He was a laborer, working in the meat-packing plants. He died in '92, pretty young. Well, he was relatively young, in his 60s. My mom is still living; she's 82. She was born in Chicago. Her parents came from Mexico at the turn of the century, about 1917, 1918. They worked in the factories here in the city. My grandmother was a housewife; she kept the house while her husband worked. She would do things that were homey, like cook food and stuff like that. My grandfather worked in the stackyards all his life until he died. He died early, as well—in his 60s. I have three blood brothers, direct brothers; I have a half-brother; I have a step-brother; then I have four sisters and a step-sister—a pretty large family.

My family is really my gay friends. I love my blood family, but so much of my life has been around not discussing my identity, up until recently. I've always been a part of my family, but in the periphery. Now they are aware of my sexuality, but I think even when I was going through this process, they were aware. It was the military policy: "Don't ask; don't tell." I have probably one sister that I'm very close to now, because she has scleroderma, a skin disease, so I've been helping her a lot. I own a condo and she stays there. She's watching it for me. She helps me out; I help her out. I've helped her out with her medical stuff, too. She's been the one person I've spoken with the most about me and my life; she knows my partner.

I do research for living. I've been doing that for 20-something years, since 1987. During that period, I've been in and out of graduate school and I'm finally finishing this year. Hopefully, that will put me further into the researcher role, but I'm tired of doing this stuff. Sometimes I want to change. I don't know. If I had to do it again, I would do something different—be a carpenter or something very manual, where I could see the product. I do that at home now and it's peaceful; it's very calming to me.

My first awareness of my sexuality was a kind of sexual interaction with a friend of mine in my neighborhood. I was 18 years old and out of high school. I was kind of late at my awareness about sex compared with some people. I had feelings for men before then, but I wasn't aware of what it meant; I probably denied it. We were the typical—you get drunk, you end up in the same house, and it gets sexual. I enjoyed it, but I remember the next day feeling shame. My friend actually wanted to talk about it, but I didn't. It wasn't until college that I became more active. It's been more and more self-discovery about what it's about being gay, but also with respect to my family. I never talked to them about it. This was all kind of secret, secret behavior. I was at school, so sex occurred there, or else at friends' homes, college friends who were gay. And actually they were African American.

I came from a neighborhood that was Latino, but in the university there were about 14 Latino students among the graduate and the undergraduate schools. So, I gravitated toward the African American community because they accepted me. I was different; I was not in the dominant Anglo culture. That is who I hung out with in terms of dinner and lunch. We had a little circle of men that were coming out.

There was a lot of stigma around homosexuality, and I had friends who left school for that. They had emotional issues because they were labeled faggots. Our behavior was pretty much undercover. We would go into the city; my friends took me out and exposed me to the gay community on Chicago's North Side. Back then, there were big disco bars. It was 1970 and it was fabulous. I remember loving it because they were people like me.

I was always a student. I always had that protective identity. I was the first person to go to college in my family, so they were proud of that, but they knew that I was different from them. I had a very working-class family. I knew they were proud of me going to school. Plus, at that time, my mother had left; she left us with our grandmother. We were much separated. There wasn't a lot of inquiry into what I was doing, as long was my life was going OK (that's what my dad would tell me).

I told one of my sisters that I was gay after I graduated from college. Her reaction was to cry.

"Why are you crying?" I asked.

She said, "I didn't realize you were holding this in for so long and having such a tough life."

I replied, "Actually, I'm enjoying it, so don't cry."

Her reaction kind of took me back a little bit. I didn't tell anyone again for years, until my dad died. I decided at that point I was going to tell my mom. I didn't want her to die and not know, and I told her. But my mom never asked me anything more, she still—to this day—rarely asks me about it. That is just her way of coping with it. I've had that struggle with my family: knowing versus taking it in.

I've done therapy for years. I kind of reached a realization, after talking to my therapist about it over the years, that I'm expecting my family to acknowledge my sexual orientation, but they live in a heteronormative world. They don't know how to approach someone, besides just loving them as their brother or son. Now they have met my partner (we have been together for a year and a half). They met my previous partner, too, but this is the first time it is all open. My current partner is very gregarious and it's made me more comfortable too, actually, even though he isn't totally out with his family—so weird. It's just a different level of support I feel with this particular partner. I ended up making a decision last year; I brought him to my nephew's wedding.

My partner has his own issues with his family and he decided to tackle them as well. I met his mother and his brothers, and they were very gracious to me. His mom loves me; we get along very well. This relationship is different; it's very special to me. He is 43, a bit younger than me. Quite a bit younger!

Now we hold hands on Michigan Avenue; we kiss each other. We went to the movies in the park last year. The environment there was very neutral and people were very not supportive, but they don't care. During the movie, he'd be laying in my lap and people didn't say anything. We were walking away from there one night last year and some young kids (and they tend to be young teenager types) pulled their car over. We were walking hand in hand and they yelled some bullshit. I had a bottle and I wanted to throw it. My partner said, "Let's just keep going." I thought about it for 2 or 3 days. It was just burning me up.

This relationship has been kind of liberating for me. I'm being out and all of a sudden see this kind of social reality. A few weeks ago, I was riding my bike home and there is nothing particularly gay about that, except that I'm an outsider to the community. People yelled at me, "Fucking bitch!" because I'm not black. I guess I had a nice outfit on or something. Anyone who isn't kind of "gangish," they see it as anti-male.

When I was younger, I learned people's stories of their homophobia in the black community and they taught me how to navigate college safely. There are continuous warning signs about how you express yourself that might provoke a violent incident. It makes me think, "Why do I have to go through this?" I'm 56 years old. That is why people end up moving into the gay community or into a more supportive environment, because you get tired of it. It gets irritating.

I think of myself as a Latino. I use that general category and I'll give you my reason why. During my high school days, I went to a high school that was in a poor community on the South Side of Chicago. It was equally mixed between black, white, Mexican, and Puerto Rican. When I was growing up, there was a lot of conflict between Puerto Riçans and Mexicans. There was a lot of turmoil between whites and blacks, and a lot of black students were fighting for rights in class and for recognition of the civil rights movement. The Latino students organized. We were going against the belief that Mexicans and Puerto Ricans had a natural antagonism. We were asking for a Latino curriculum in school. By that time, teachers were tired of hearing it from the black students. We were asking for history—Puerto Rican and Mexican history in class. So, I took that kind of identity as a statement against divisions between Latinos, as kind of more unified. We have uniqueness, but as far as the dominant culture went, we needed to maintain a unified stance.

Right now my social network is mostly African American, then white, with minimal Latino. Growing up, my neighborhood was probably 80% to 90% Latino. They were second- and third-generation immigrants, very acculturated, but working class. We had a few white friends, but they were outsiders. They were the ones who had to struggle to get accepted into the group. So it was different. That's all I knew. I had all the stereotypes about African Americans: they're very dangerous and bad. That's all everyone knew. That's the history of Chicago, the way you were taught about different neighborhoods.

My first experience with African Americans was in high school. I ended up having a few friends, but I hung out mostly with my friends from my neighborhood. College, again, was a different thing because we were within a university that was predominantly white, so minorities tended to clump together for support. The African American community was very open and willing to accept me. That shaped my life from that point—my attraction, my friendships, and my knowledge.

The first time I became aware of AIDS was when one of my good friends that I went to high school with (he was probably my best friend), ended up becoming positive. He was in Washington, DC. That was 1984 or '83. I was scared in the sense that it was mysterious. It had that stigma of being mysterious—no cure. I probably was one of the most promiscuous people you can imagine. I knew, without being an epidemiologist, "OK, it's in New York and San Francisco. I've just got to be careful." My friend died in '85. That was early on in the epidemic.

I have a lot of friends who have died from AIDS. I have that personal loss. With this friend of mine, I remember him dying and him being a leader. He was one of the first people, one of the first African Americans, to put himself out there publicly and be involved in national-level work, trying to confront stigma, really early on. I saw him deteriorate. I also remember going to Mexico to get medication that they didn't sell here because it was experimental. It didn't help him.

I remember my first really physical fear of HIV/AIDS was with him. Maybe the last 2 months of his life, he had been hospitalized and wanted to go home. He was tired of being in the hospital. When he got discharged, I met him at the hospital, we got in a cab, and we went to his house. There were boxes and a bed not made up. I was there to take care of him for maybe 4 days. It was my job; I told him I'd do it. I remember feeling uncomfortable touching him and cleaning up his bathroom where he had been a few days before he was hospitalized; it was nasty. I was afraid to clean it, but I did.

I would have to take breaks and leave the house because he was very irritable and demanding. He was powerless.

One time, he looked so sad. He was in his bed and I was cleaning up. He was in physical pain and wanted his little stuffed bunny. He used to be a big muscular guy, and then he was frail and wanted his bunny. I saw him just holding it and it just made me go hold him. That's when I made a decision to get over my fears. I thought, "Oh my God! This person is going through this and I can't be afraid to hold him." That was my confrontation. I took all the precautions I needed to, but I cannot not be human.

That experience is what got me into the field of HIV research and prevention. Those experiences made me realize I need to do something. Since then, I've seen a lot of other friends go—very good friends. It just made me more resolute about my own health. I knew early on that medications weren't working, so I didn't want to be tested.

A lot of these friends who died, I call them *warriors* because they fought that early battle and they taught me a lot. I'd say to myself, "If I'm positive, I'm going to know what to do," because I saw them deal with their own personal adversity, dealing with their families, relationships, loneliness, and health issues. So, when I finally did get tested, it was right after HAARTs [highly active antiretroviral therapies] came out. It was '98, because one of my last really good friends had died right before; he decided to take his life. (I had two friends take their lives.) He consciously made that decision: "I'm tired of this." He had been infected since he was 19 and he was 30-something already. He just got tired of medications. He made that decision to stop taking anything; he went really quickly. I talked to him about me getting tested and he was a really good support for me.

When I got my positive result, I remember the woman said, "You are dealing with this very well."

"Because I have a lot of good friends who have gone through this," I replied.

She asked, "Are you going to be okay?"

I said, "Actually, I am. I have a real good support system." My friends' doctors became my doctors; all the stuff my friends went through was a learning experience for me.

My health is very good now. My first setback was right after I became positive. The doctor put me on a regimen and I had an immediate negative reaction. I got deadly ill. None of my friends went through it. Well, they went through it but they were long-term survivors; they had been through a million of regimes already. I stopped for 1 month, took another regimen, and have never had any problems since then. Since '98, my T-cell counts have always been very high, so maybe I have a weak strain or maybe it was a recent infection.

I have cholesterol issues. I'm on Lipitor; that's my only problem with this—well, I shouldn't say *only* because I swear this medication has a side effect that makes you drag. It takes me until 11 o'clock in the morning to get up, to feel vibrant. So sometimes I feel like stopping. I feel like I'm tired of taking it. I talked with a good friend of mine who is younger and really smart in terms of looking up stuff. We always talk about new developments out there. I'm ready for the next new thing.

As far as the health issues, if it wasn't for those people before me, my life probably would be different. If it wasn't for my job, I would be different. I've worked in the HIV field. I'm lucky because I have access to resources and know where to go. I have my own mental health issues that I deal with from my family life.

I do what's called *cognitive restructuring*. If something is making me feel bad, I think about what is making me feel this way and I try to change the feeling. It's the idea that you feel the way that you think. I ask myself, "Why am I feeling this way? I'm feeling this way because this is happening." Sometimes we tend to magnify things, so I just need to stop doing that. I have a friend who is a psychologist and she shared this with me and it's been very useful. So, I get depressed, but it doesn't last long because I look for strategies out of it. I don't think it's a personality thing, but a training thing. It's a resource that I have and I'm lucky to have access to it.

I'm thinking that I'm getting old. I know I'm getting old! I get sad sometimes thinking about it. Now I'm in the mode of "OK, I got to prepare." Part of it has been to talk with my family about my identity. The next is to work with my partner to see if our relationship is going to go anywhere. "OK, we've been together a year and 4 months." I said, "I'm gonna give it a year and a half, and I'm pushing; I've already pushed a little." I want to spend my life, the reminder of my life, in a supportive environment with someone, to help each other. "So, are we going to do this or not?" If not, then I'll just move on, which I would hate, because I really care about this person, but he's coming around, even though he is younger. I'm thinking about it that way. I want to get a partner and I want to be able to have someone to rely on to share a life with so that we can take care of each other.

I have a small community of friends. I don't have that many really close friends here in Chicago, very few. A lot of my friends are on the East Coast. There are a couple of them who are happy, but they are kind of relegated to not being in a relationship. A relationship is important to me; I don't know why. My East Coast friends are around my age. They think they'll never get a relationship, so they are developing the remainder of their years around how to be happy and not in a relationship. But I know I'm not going to be happy that way, for whatever reason. As I said, a relationship is important to me, so I'm working to try to develop it. And I think, "What if my illness. . . ?" Who knows? I hope nothing happens, but what if something happens? I want someone to be there for me. I don't see myself with my family. I love my family, but we've gone different ways. I don't think I would be happy alone. I really don't.

The other issue—and I run across this so much—if we are going to rely on the gay community, which I don't think I do, is the whole youth and aging thing. As you get older, you lose attraction. There are a lot of guys my age that aren't in relationships. Sometimes when I go out with my partner, I see them. They are still into the idea that you find a relationship in a bar, and I guess, for me, life is about building affirmative relationships, and I'm putting my own values on it. Some people don't care about that. This buddy of mine on the East Coast, he turned 60 and he's happy. But I can tell sometimes that he is sad because he is not in a relationship. He's resigned that he is not going to be in a relationship, and I know that he messes around. He goes out and picks up men in the trees. He is a man; he has a sexual drive. Again, maybe I'm putting a value on his sexual activity; I don't know.

Building affirmative relationships is all tied with identity. Then there is a whole group of men, older black men, who are still in heterosexual relationships because there is some security in that for them. They've been in them forever and they are not going to get out of them. They have responsibilities and they have informal agreements with their female partners, like, "Well, you go out and do what you're going to do."

I have excellent healthcare because of my job. I get really good benefits. It costs me more, but I have a really good doctor, medications are paid, so that's great. I am a member of health club; I try to do that to stay fit. That's the other thing that I know I have to do to keep my health, I figure. My boyfriend is big; he's a little bit overweight (he even says that about himself) and he's younger than me. But he has health issues—not HIV, but he's had a stroke, he broke his leg in a couple of places, and has a family history of high blood pressure. He has more health issues than me.

I wouldn't mind getting into teaching, even if it's part-time. Actually, I always talk with my partner about doing something together, like a business. I'm thinking of leaving the field, maybe, or after I retire. I'm interested in doing something creative. We talked about a restaurant, and I know those things are very difficult. The failure rate is very high, but the positive is that I'm energized; he's energized. I'm lucky enough to be able to have access to resources and know where to look, not that that guarantees anything, but it puts me ahead of other people. I think that would help solidify our relationship and kind of help us build something. So that's another goal.

I also think of community, like building a small community, understanding that a component of it has to be geographic as well. The Internet and phones are good, but

I want to be able to have a real community to go to physically and spend time with people, and have people close to me—live in the same area, the same building. It would be nice to buy a building where everyone knows each other. Get a big building, everyone pitch in, and there's your community. It doesn't all have to be gay people. It can be family; it can be people who are supportive of each other.

It's weird that I'm finally finishing my dissertation. A lot of people haven't done that. My neighborhood? Probably no one. My family? I'll be the first. I'm proud of that. I'm very proud of working in this field. I feel I have had an impact on the community. I got good friends, very good friends, very supportive for the most part. And I think my parents raised me right, even though they were divorced and this and that.

GRAND

"I Am a Humanitarian"

I'M 65 YEARS OLD AND WAS born in Mississippi. I work for a social services agency on the South and West sides of Chicago. Have done it for 20 years. My mother and father both are deceased. I have one brother still alive, lost one brother to drugs, and two brothers who are deceased. I have three sisters who are still alive. I have two sons and two grand sons.

On this side of town, you don't want to be thought of as being old, so you do things to keep yourself young. I have a friend who is 18 years younger than me. We've been together about 7½ years. He is bisexual, so we have an open relationship. We are planning on having a house in the suburbs for more privacy in terms of our lifestyle, particularly because of my public profile. My family knows about my lifestyle, but his family doesn't know about his lifestyle. He's got two kids, 17 and 19 years old. I'm like a godfather to his kids.

I went through treatment for prostate cancer the past couple of years; it's in remission. It turned my life upside down in the process. At one time I weighed 355. I'm down to 300 now. Another 40 to 45 lb I want to lose, to get down to 255. I've become kind of sedentary, working on a computer day in and day out. I do a lot of reading and writing. I remember one day thinking to myself, "Don't you have a social life? You are always at the computer! Yeah, but I got to get this done." I'm kind of a hands-on CEO.

I have a master's in administration. I was trying to work on my doctorate, but decided I was not going to teach in college; I wasn't interested in it. I am a humanitarian. One day, a young guy who was strung out on drugs—at that time we didn't know about AIDS—approached me for help. I was also approached to take on some homeless persons because I had a large house. I took in a couple of people and all of a sudden I went from having 2 to 10 staff persons. I started detailing how to put a transitional house, or a recovery home, together. I put the whole thing together and gradually built it into a few-million-dollars organization, providing the whole gamut of social services. Many of the guys adopted me as a second father, so that required I carry a certain image. Many knew about my lifestyle, but I kept it private, a separate part. They respected that. It has worked well, it served me well, and if I had my life to do over again, I would do the same thing over again.

I don't remember too much about the Deep South. I remember my parents headed north. I went to a Catholic elementary school. When I started first grade, I was moved to the third grade. I was an altar boy. I was the only black in my class, so I went through the hardships of discrimination and all the stuff like that. I kind of suppressed my academic ability because when I scored high, I would set the curve for the class, and that created a problem. And there was always a fight. Oh man, I went through hell.

I was the top student in the class and got a scholarship to go to college. I went to a private college and played basketball there. Again, I was the only black there. I did very well academically, but it was one thing to live in your cultural community and another to live in the white academic world. I went to school up on the North Side of Chicago and I would go home. My speech set me apart from everybody here in my home community. They used to call me "professor." Trying to mix and blend in was not easy, and trying to mix and blend on the other side wasn't easy. I dropped out and went to a junior college. Then I went back to the university and got my bachelor's degree in education. I became a teacher in an elementary school at 17. I didn't really think about how young I was as much as I thought about what I could do for these kids. I was an idealist; I really wanted to help these kids.

I even surprised myself, how well I did. I come from a large family—there were nine of us—and I was the oldest. I had to help raise my brothers and sisters. My dad worked for a condominium building. We had to get up in the morning at 5 o'clock to go shovel coal and put it in the furnace.

My dad said, "This is what you will be doing."

I recall telling him, "Pop, I don't want to be a janitor. I don't want to do this." "Pop, I can't do this. I want to go to school." "I love you, Pop, but I don't want to do this." I saw that hurt look on his face and I felt so bad. "I don't want to do this for the rest of my life," I said. "I want to do something with my life." At the time, I explained to him what I wanted to do: I wanted to teach. As a kid I wanted to teach and train people and do things with people. I got into teaching. I still lived at home. In fact, I lived at home until I got married, when I was 20 or 21.

Before I got married, I was in the park one day and someone called to me, "You gay." It startled me and intrigued me. I looked and I said, "Is there something that I'm doing that makes you feel that I'm like that?" I thought, "Do I show?" It really bothered me. And that was the determining question that led me to get married.

I did not want to be what is now known as a *drag queen*. "I don't want to do that." I was having fantasies about other men and, of course, there was nobody to talk to about being gay. I lived my life in that closet, all those years. Until one day, when I was teaching in high school on the West Side of Chicago and there was another guy there.

He came to me one day and said, "I'd like to talk to you." We had lunch and he asked me, "Do you know who you are?"

"What the hell are you talking about?" I asked. Do I know who I am? Yeah, I know who I am!" I wasn't married at the time. It's like he saw something in me that I did not know was there.

He said, "What you need to do is to go find yourself, because you are searching for yourself." He said, "You understand me. You don't want to admit it."

He sent me to a club called the Cellar. So I went and ordered some orange juice, because I didn't drink. I just watched the people. It was like going to the movies—fascinating. I was scared to death!

One guy, an older guy, walked in. He said, "Do not get involved with anybody here unless you come to me and you talk to me. You are young and you really don't know who you are." Then he said, "I want you to go to the club Normandy and I want you to go in and look and see who you are."

I went, but I didn't go in. I looked through the door and I saw kissing, hugging, and everything else. After that I said,

"That's not who I am. It's not who I want to be." And yet, there was feeling inside me that said, "You may need to examine who you are. Maybe they see something in you that you don't see." That's kind of where I went. That gave me enough courage to go through the experience with someone older, who walked me through the process, the male part of the process, initially. And I went from that process to becoming and playing the female role in the process, which I do now. It's been like that for the past 40 years. Forty years with no women.

When I got married, I had two kids born within the first 3 years. And then it was like, "I love my kids!" But I wanted out of the relationship because I didn't love my wife. I married her to get out of the house. I married because I wanted grandkids. I married her for all the wrong reasons. I had two great kids. Suffice it to say, if I could do it over again, I would do the same thing—maybe a little different in some things.

I always kept my private life away from my work (the agency), so that no one could ever say, "Oh I saw him in this. I saw him in that." Even now, to this day, they couldn't tell you that they saw me here or there. I'm just a private person to that extent.

We came from a very poor family. My mother was the driving force in the family. She instilled the competitiveness in us from almost day one: "You got to be good." "You got to get it." "You got to go to the best schools." "You got to work hard." She instilled that work ethic in us. I remember helping my brother with his homework because he was real slow. The other brother was very quick academically; my sisters were all quick academically. Everybody graduated, but that one brother got involved in drugs. I lost my brothers to drugs. Ironically, I lost three brothers—to drugs and AIDS. My older sister came out real bad; she's gay. She ended up going to the penitentiary. She found God while she was there. Now she's doing very well, raising four kids—my brother's grandkids. My youngest sister gave my second sister her two kids to take care of, and she put the kids through school.

I wanted to become a priest. I told God that if I won a college scholarship, I would follow the outside world; if I didn't win the scholarship, I would become a priest. When I got that scholarship it was like saying, "God does not want you to become a priest; he's got other things planned for you." My whole life has been built around that concept: God didn't bring me this far to let me down. He's got something for me to do.

People ask, "How can you be gay and be Catholic at the same time?" Easy! God does not favor one relationship over another. I truly believe that. I believe that each individual has to stand before the Almighty and give an account of himself.

God weighs like the scales of justice, and weighs what you do, what you did wrong, and makes a conscious decision: "You did some bad stuff, but when I look at the overall picture of your life, you did a great deal for a whole lot of people. How can I discount that? While you guys down there may not consider your sins and this and the other, that's not how I look at it. I look at it radically different. You cannot begin to comprehend how I view your life."

I think sometimes we get so preoccupied with religion, and we destroy people in the name of religion.

Nowadays I don't go to church on Sunday as I should. I wake up on Sunday morning and think, "I'm gonna work in your vineyard today."

God's probably cursing me out, saying, "Today is *my* day. You supposed to come to church on Sunday."

I think to myself, "God, I can do more working over here in the vineyard than sitting in a chair listening to somebody who doesn't believe what he says himself." I feel pretty guilty about that. If I have one thing to answer for, that is that I don't go to Church on Sunday.

I remember when I was very young, though, I went to the South with my family on vacation one summer. I was 7, 8, or maybe 9 years of age. Never will forget. This is Memphis, Tennessee. Cousins took me to the store and I asked for some cookies or something. I put them on the counter and I think the clerk said, "OK, is that all?"

I said, "Yeah, that's all."

My cousins told me, "You're supposed to say 'yes, sir.' "

I looked at my cousins and asked, "Why?"

"Because you're supposed to," they said.

Again, I asked, "Why?"

"Because you're black."

I shrugged my shoulders. Then we got outside and my cousin said, "Do you know you can get killed for that?"

AIDS turned my life completely upside down because, at the time, I was very promiscuous. After AIDS, all the promiscuity stopped. Period. It just stopped. I hadn't taken on a lover per se—one nighters, AIDS stopped me cold. "I cannot afford—I don't know who has it; I don't know who has transmitted it."

By then I had started to take in the homeless, and I never will forget one guy who was sitting down on the corner and I asked him, "Why are you sitting down there?"

He was crying and he said, "I want to go home."

I asked, "Why can't you go home?"

"I can't tell you."

I said, "Why can't you? What did you do? Did you kill somebody?"

He said, "No."

I just kept at it, and he said, "I'm sick."

And I said, "Oh, God. Man, come here, come here." He came to me and I put my arms around him. "It's going to be alright. You are going to be alright. You're going to be healed."

There were others who came in, and gradually I learned what was occurring—a lot of sad experiences. We had a lot of guys who were dying because they would go from HIV to AIDS.

Through that whole period of time I was scared to death, but at the same time I felt like if God had not wanted me to be in this business, then I would be dead too. I would have contracted AIDS. There were many days that I cried with them, trying to help them walk through—. Watching them die, helping set up funerals, it took a toll on me, to say the least. And to this day, it does. It took a toll on me. So much so that when my brothers died, I backed away from helping anybody with HIV for a couple of years. Most of the guys were straight; they weren't gay. At that time, everybody in my home was family. When you come to our agency, we are family; we look out for one another.

Early on, I took precautions: safe sex. I would do things to limit the exposure. I would not give anybody a blow job; if it was anal sex, it was with a condom. I took those precautions early. Even to this day, I'm not sleeping with anyone, except my partner, and he feels good about it.

He has a house in the suburbs. For a long time, he was content with the norm of family, then all of a sudden he came to live with me. But I was living in a house with the guys, so we kept a safe, discreet distance. I took him to work every day and picked him up every day, until he got his car. So we kindled the warm relationship that we had initially after he moved out. But now, we call each other every morning. We talk; that's our morning. As I said, he is 18 years younger than me. He is a cook; he likes to be around me. I'm his surrogate father. He calls me "Pop."

I have anxiety attacks because my partner has a flip side to life. I wonder in my mind how far our relationship going to last. "Is he going to get hooked up with somebody that he is going to want to go with, stay with, and leave you?" That is a constant worry. We have been together more than 7 years.

I have an HIV test every 6 months, even though I'm not sexually active. But, I have it every 6 months. I'm fine. I don't smoke, I don't do drugs. I have a couple of drinks once a week or something. My doctor saw an elevation in my PSA (prostate-specific antigen) count and he said, "We got to watch it."

I went through the whole process, the biopsy, and all that kind of stuff. Then, for a period of 4 or 6 months, it rose again—the onset of second stage. The doctor sent me to an oncologist. The first oncologist and I didn't get along too well because what he wanted, I didn't want. My doctor sent me to a different oncologist. For the past 2 years I've been going to see him and he's been taking good care of me.

He's a really nice guy. I went through initial radiation and a couple of months beyond that I started bleeding. One day he discovered that I had lost a half a liter of blood.

He said he knew what was causing it. "When you went through radiation, there was some collateral damage, and it takes a long time for it to heal."

They put me into a hyperbaric oxygen chamber. I went through that for about 4 months. When they did get it fixed, they wanted me to come back for the last 15 sessions. So I did my 30 sessions. Actually, I think I wound up doing 45, 50 sessions. I receive home healthcare, too. The therapist comes out every week to check blood pressure, all the vitals, heart, lungs.

"You're cool. You're fine."

My blood pressure, average, is about 120 to 130 every week.

I want to travel. In fact, we are saving some money to travel to New Orleans this summer. My friend has money and he wants to travel, "Hell, let's go!" He wants to leave his job.

I said, "Wait until we do what we do. Let's put this piece together first, so that we will be financially stable. Then let's hit it! Let's get a van and let's just go."

So we might do some traveling this year.

I have a passion for this: working with the people I work with. It's something that I don't see leaving in the foreseeable future. I'm training my son to take on the responsibilities, and I'm training my friend to take on a for-profit entity and am working with him in setting up a housing program. I want to see if I can bridge between the two to help them hold it all together. So I don't see retirement. I'm not on that page. I couldn't even begin doing retirement. I'd go crazy.

I've been able to make a difference. I'm not the most loved guy when it gets to certain things with the politicians. They call me a nonconformist because I do things others wouldn't. I've been around for a long time; I've been here for a while. I just have a lot of respect for what I've done and what I've accomplished. Then, when I look at the number of people who I have helped and the number of people who come back—.

Just like today, one of the guys, a street vendor down the street, looked at me and said, "You don't know me?" He said, "I saw you a couple of mornings and I wanted to say something but I wasn't sure it was you." He told me, "I have grown kids now, four kids."

Things like that make me feel good. And see how well all the people who come to our recovery center are doing. Some of them have started their own programs. One guy became a psychologist; another one, a doctor. I guess with Facebook, now there are a whole lot of folks that say, "Oh, there you are!" It makes you feel good. It does.

I'm self-reliant. I grew up being self-reliant. There were some happy days; there were some sad days, but there was a lot of happiness. We were pioneers in some of the stuff that we did. I just wish I could have done more. On the flip side, had I been more of a conformist, I probably could have accomplished more.

CHARLIE

"Being Older and Being by Yourself"

I'M 56. I GREW UP IN CHICAGO, originally on the West Side. My family moved out to the suburbs when I was a kid. I work now as a computer analyst. I have been doing this work for the past 10 years. I have a master's degree in social work. I don't have a formal degree in computer sciences. My degree is in social work, but I wanted to do something different, and I guess I wanted to make some money. My background as a social worker is actually as a community organizer. I did community organizing in Chicago and then in El Salvador. On the West Side of Chicago I made very little money and in El Salvador I didn't get paid at all. So, I wanted to do something where I actually had a salary.

I'm bilingual: English and Spanish. I worked in Humboldt Park for a community group that probably 70% of the clients were Hispanic—mostly Puerto Rican, some Mexican. We built lawn composting, we did housing co-ops, tenant-run housing, and things like that. I was actually in charge of property management; it was pretty imperative that I learn to speak Spanish. People would come to me with a problem and they wanted to talk to me confidentially. They didn't want to talk to me through a translator.

When I think about age, I think, particularly thinking about myself and aging, I think two things: one is, "What else do I want to do with my life?" That's one of the reasons why I left social work, because I wanted to have other experiences. I still think that there are other kinds of careers, other places I want to live, things I want to do that I haven't had time to do, or that I want to do before I get too old. The other thing is, I'm still single. Well, I'm single again. And, as you get older, I think that is not a situation that I want to see continue. So that is a concern: being older and being by yourself. I have lots of friends. I'm real active in a lot of organizations, but I just think, at the end of the day, I don't want to be by myself all the time.

As a kid I was always different. I don't mean just different in the sense that I was gay, because I don't think I knew what that meant back then. I was different in the sense that I came from a family where both my parents were professionals, but we lived in a working-class neighborhood. I was different in the sense that my family had different values. I didn't do a lot of things other kids did, because it was always impressed upon us that we had to be really good in school and study. I took music lessons after school and I went to religious school after regular school. So I was just different than other kids. Also, I am Jewish. I grew up in a neighborhood that was predominantly not Jewish; there were very few Jewish kids. I think that's the one thing that sticks out: that I was different.

My mother was a violinist; she's still a violinist, actually. She's 80. She still teaches and performs. My father was a chemist. My father died when I was 19. And I have two brothers. My parents were very involved. They put a lot of emphasis on education. They also put a lot of emphasis on organized activities, and things like that. We took piano lessons, we took religious school, we were involved in Boy Scouts, and they were very active. They supervised stuff. They volunteered stuff. My mom was PTA president, and Cub Scout leader, and all kinds of things like that.

I think the thing was, again, I felt different. There weren't many Jewish kids in my neighborhood, and the few Jewish kids there were sort of like me, in the sense that their parents were professionals in a working-class neighborhood. I didn't feel any sense of discrimination or anything like that, but you definitely kind of felt like, "Oh, the Jewish kids were the smart kids." I don't think people looked down upon us. It wasn't like people were anti-Semitic; if they were, I didn't pick up on it.

I didn't have a lot of the fun that other kids did. I didn't join sports or anything like that. I played the piano a lot. As I said, I was in Cub Scouts and Boys Scouts. I had my own little group of friends.

The one thing that stands out is, this was the Vietnam War era, and I was real active in political things. Here again, I lived in a working-class neighborhood, suburban neighborhood in Chicago, fairly conservative neighborhood, fairly Republican, and being antiwar, having long hair, and participating in antiwar rallies did not make me really popular.

I would say I went to rallies probably as early as 13 or 14. A lot of stuff was going on in the city. My parents would generally not let me go, although I did. When I started high school, probably 13 or 14, I was in a citywide Jewish youth organization. We used to have our meetings in downtown Chicago, which meant after school, twice a month, I got to take the train downtown and come home late. There were Jewish kids from all over the city. I think that's where I got a lot of my antiwar inspiration, from the other kids that I met. Most of these kids would have lived in the big Jewish neighborhoods in the city, in the far North Side. Those neighborhoods were a lot more liberal, a lot more progressive. We were involved in some antiwar organizing—rallies, marches, other political sorts of things. I remember there was this movement called Hike for the Hungry, which at the time was—I mean, now everybody does walks; you are walking for this, you are walking for that. This is, like, almost 40 years ago. So I had to organize a local group for what was called Hike for the Hungry, which at the time was a huge thing. It was the first time I've ever put something together like this and there were literally tens of thousands of mostly high school kids all over the city who did this. It was a bunch of long-hair, want-to-be hippies.

To me, it all seemed like it made sense, and to my friends and stuff it made sense, and then I was surprised to find out that I had neighbors who thought it was just this horribly radical idea. I remember going to one neighbor's house, and I knew they were fundamentalist Christians, but it didn't really sink in to me what that meant until I went and talked with them. Part of it was just going around the neighborhood and getting pledges from people. I went and talked to my neighbors. I thought it was great that my neighbors, of course—they'd support me. I was really shocked that they started asking all these questions like this was some communist sort of thing: "How do we know where this money is going?" "Isn't the money going to some Communist Party or something?" It just sort of shocked me that they would even think that. Maybe I was just totally naive, but I just had this idea: "Oh, we are just helping needy people."

Most of my friends in high school were Jewish, even though they were a small minority in the school. I mean, I just knew I was different. I knew I didn't do a lot of the other things kids do. I didn't do sports. I didn't like sports. I didn't date much. Well, I didn't date at all. It wasn't something I was very interested in. But if the question is, "Did I think I was different because I was gay?" I don't think I'd figured that out yet.

I had my group of friends and we were pretty close and I was accepted by them. At that time, when living in a very politicized environment because of the war, there was so much tension. There were people that put me down. In my mind, the world was in two camps: there were the good guys, who believed in all these causes and were antiwar, and there were the bad guys. So there were definitely people in our neighborhood who hated us because we were protesting or because we had long hair.

Once I went to college, things changed. I went to college when I was—actually, I was 17 when I started college. It was a fun experience. Looking back on it, it wasn't just partying, but it wasn't really serious academics either. I don't think a lot of people study real hard. I don't think we were really studying.

I went out with a few people and obviously it was the first time I was going out with guys, but I didn't have a boyfriend or anything per se. Actually, it's kind of an amusing story. I was probably a sophomore, and still very naive and innocent. I remember we were at a party and this girl was, like, really, really drunk. She was just like flirting with me incredibly and I couldn't figure out what she wanted. She was clearly trying to pick me up and trying to get me to take her home. Eventually, I did, but she practically had to hit me over the head to tell me this is what she wanted: "Oh, God! I'm so drunk I don't know what I'm doing, and I'm all alone because my roommate is gone away for the weekend." I couldn't figure out why she kept saying that to me. The funny part of the story is that she had been going out with this other guy, who I knew, and I thought she was going out with him. Then I found out that evening that they were no longer going out. Long story short, I ended up back at her room with her and it was not the most successful evening. Afterward, this other guy that she had been going out with found out what had happened and came to talk to me about it. It turned out that the reason he was no longer going out with her was because he decided he was gay. He told me; he invited me back to his place. We both went to her wedding about 4 years later. It was kind of amusing.

The other thing going on was that there were a lot of people in my dorm who were very openly gay, both students and faculty. Probably wasn't as big a shock. I think in high school I didn't even know that it existed. Again, this is 40 years ago. I think a couple of years prior to this I would have been totally freaked out because I didn't know. I knew what the word meant, but I didn't know anybody who was like that and I thought everybody who was like that was weird or effeminate. But the guys who were openly gay were not the stereotype of what, at the time, I might have thought gay people were like: effeminate and flamboyant.

My mom, she's 80 now, is very friendly and supportive and accepting, but she just doesn't want to hear about stuff. It's not that she doesn't want to hear. It's that she doesn't want to talk about stuff, and it's not just gay stuff. She doesn't want to hear about my brothers' personal life. She just doesn't think it's proper. But, when I have gone out with people in the past, she met them and she was very supportive. She always said, "Do you want to bring so-and-so over for dinner?"

I remember when I was in my 20s and I was going out with this guy who was an accountant. I was, at the time, a community organizer, so I still had long hair, dirty blue jeans, and t-shirts. We had to go to something at the synagogue, so I showed up wearing a really nice suit.

My mom was like, "Oh! That's a really nice suit, does that belong to—?"

So I was like, "Yeah." And actually it did.

When HIV came, I was in Chicago working on the West Side. I remember being pretty scared, partly because I had the environment in my 20s in the '70s, when I went back to Chicago and just out of the closet. Things were pretty wild. People fooled around a lot. People went to the bar and did things in the backroom, sometimes in the front room in the bar. It was a bit scary because you didn't know. We didn't know very much at all at the time. We didn't know what caused it, we didn't know what prevented it, we didn't know what was safe and safer. "Could you get it from kissing someone?" I mean, who knew? Then, my roommate from college, who never came out to me, all of a sudden got AIDS and I was like, "How did it happen?" He was, like, 27 years old and he had AIDS. He died. He was 27, 28 years old and he died of AIDS and there was no treatment or cure or anything. That was sort of the reality then: you got AIDS, there's nothing they can do for you, and that was it.

I remember there was a lot of paranoia. Things changed, from initially not having a clue what it was or where it came from or how to prevent it, to starting to talk about safer sex and things you could do. But it was scary. It was depressing. When they first started having a test a lot of people would not get tested because there was no treatment, and people thought they just didn't want to know. Then AZT came out and that was not great, but it was something. Little by little, it got better and better. It got to the point where eventually people were actually able to live.

It's curious, though, coming forward now to where we are at now. People I know who are my age and older, I think still live with this idea firmly implanted in their minds that you always have to be safe if you are not in a monogamous relationship. I know a lot of people who are younger who don't have this idea anymore, who just have this idea: "Oh yeah, well there's medication and it's not going to kill you." People in my generation know; it's been ingrained in our head. People we knew died when they were in their 20s and 30s. People we knew were horribly sick before they died. They had a horrible death at age 27.

It's been a long time. I think, at the time, I sort of felt like—. Initially I thought, for sure, sooner or later, I would find out that I had AIDS. When I didn't, I started getting tested on a regular basis, and testing seemed to have a purpose because there were things you could do if you found out you were positive. Then I started feeling like—. There is this thing they talk about: survivor guilt. In the Jewish community, people who survived the Holocaust, there's this thing called *survivor guilt*. "Why did I survive and other people die?"

I kind of almost feel like that. "How come so-and-so got it and I didn't?"

I think now, it's been so long, I kind of have moved on. To be really honest, if I think about my behavior in my 20s, statistically I should have gotten AIDS. I think some people's immune systems are different than others and I just happen to be lucky in that sense.

Nowadays life is good, in the sense that I have a lot of friends and am involved in a lot of activities that I enjoy. I think I have a decent career. I have a lot of money invested and a lot of money saved. I got good plans for the future, good prospects for the future.

I lived in Europe for several years. I have lots of friends in Europe. I was able to travel around a lot. I still have the possibility of going back to Europe. I'm just doing a lot of things that I enjoy doing. As I said before, when I was a kid, I took music lessons; now I've gotten back into that. I'm playing chamber music with a couple of people. I'm satisfied with my friendships. I'm still single. I have lots of really close friends.

I think I got into computer programming basically because I wasn't making any money as a community organizer. I don't think I ever wanted to do this for the rest of my life. It's not something like, "Oh, I've always wanted to be this when I grow up." I didn't always want to be a computer programmer. I can do it. Sometimes it's interesting, but it's not something that thrills me. It's something I can do. Sometimes it's interesting because it's challenging, but a lot of times you are doing programming for a big company. It's not something I believe in, even when I'm working for a government agency. I don't really believe in it. It's not like a cause or a purpose.

I'm at the point where I've saved enough money. I've enough money invested and, within the next year or two, I want to go back and do something that I enjoy doing. Financially, I'm in a position where I can do that without having to worry about how much I make or how much I don't make.

I've belonged to Front Runners for 15 years. We do a race to raise money for local charities. I haven't done that much lately, to be honest. When I lived in Europe I was on the board of a group that promoted alternatives to driving cars. It's probably the only sport thing I've ever done. It was sort of an easy sport because you are not actually competing. And Front Runners is a good group. I had a friend who did it. At the time, I was 40 when I joined them and I had never run in my life. It's a nice group and it's people from all different levels. Some people can't even run, some people just go walk, and others are very competitive. It's all ages. The guy that just passed away was 85 and he was still coming to Front Runners up until his 80s. There are people who are early 20s, college students—a real diverse group.

I'm involved in a couple of book groups. There's actually a book group sponsored by ALMA [the Association of Latinos/as Motivating Action, a gay men's organization] that I went to once. I might continue to go to that. This is just a chance to meet other gay people, basically, an alternative to going to bars, which I don't particularly like to do.

My health is fine, good. I've never taken medicine for anything. I'm just never sick, I guess. People tell me I should take aspirin as a preventive, but I don't. I've been a vegetarian almost 20 years. The first relationship I had, I was with a guy who was vegetarian and I always admired him and always wanted to do it, but I never got around to it. Then I went and lived in Central America, and I lived in a village that had no electricity or plumbing. What that meant was that everybody raised their own food. It was a neat kind of village. People didn't have jobs per se; everyone either hunted or farmed. People didn't really have money; they traded things. Someone would go fishing and they would come back and they would trade the fish. Someone else would cook and they would trade the food. In order to survive, everybody raised their own animals and grew their own food. I used to watch my neighbors killing animals. So that, plus I had always had this interest in becoming vegetarian anyway. Then my dad died of cancer, but my dad had lots of health problems. He was very overweight and had all kinds of chronic issues. I didn't want to end up like that. I think watching people kill animals just kind of pushed me over the edge. When I went back to Chicago, I just stopped eating meat.

My doctor is gay. I've always liked him. He's a nice guy. I've never been sick; I very rarely get sick and I very rarely need anything from a doctor other than just routine checkups.

There's this whole thing in the gay community: we are all supposed to be young and cute, and well dressed, beautiful hair, and whatever, blah, blah. I was never any of those things when I was younger. I had long hair and I didn't pay attention to how I dressed. I think you sort of feel it, though. I don't hang out in bars either, so it's not like I'm going places where I'm going to feel rejected. I hang out with my friends, but you are definitely aware that we're in a culture where there's a lot of emphasis on looks and physical appearance, and how you dress and how you wear your hair. So, as you get older, it's harder. Obviously you don't fit into the stereotypes, not that I fit into the stereotypes when I was younger, but it's much more noticeable that you don't fit in and that other people think about those things. Sometimes people don't talk to you. There's this attitude when you go into certain bars, "What are you doing here?" kind of thing. You're not supposed to talk to certain people because you are not cute enough or not good looking enough to talk to them.

In the ALMA book club, everyone there was really young. I was also the only person who wasn't Hispanic. The other book groups, two other book groups that I go to, have older guys.

Front Runners is a very friendly group, but there are definitely cute young guys, and they are friendly to a certain point. But clearly they don't talk to the old farts. We go out to eat afterward and, generally, the young people don't go or they go someplace by themselves. Part of it is, younger guys run faster, so they hang out with the people that they run with. When you get to my age, you don't run as fast.

I've done a lot of interesting things that most people haven't done. I've traveled a lot. I've been to a lot of countries and I've learned a foreign language to the point where I speak it fluently. I've done volunteer work. I did things as a community organizer that I think made a difference. I enjoy playing music. But I'm still single.

ADAM

"Age Is Just a Number; I Don't Necessarily Put Much Stock in It"

I'M 56 YEARS OLD; born and raised in Chicago. I'm a Lutheran pastor at a congregation in the suburbs. I'm open to them, open to my bishop, and open to everybody at this point in my life.

For me, age is just a number. I don't necessarily put much stock in it. I've known guys who were 56 who acted much older, acted as if their best years were behind them and this is all awful. I don't see myself in that light. I see myself as being and acting somewhat younger than the rest of my 56-year-old peers. I had a very nice celebration on my 50th birthday, but it wasn't like some kind of trauma, some kind of awful moment. It just was.

I grew up in a crazy wonderful family. My mother wasn't married. I came home to three bachelor brothers, three uncles, and a widowed aunt. I was basically raised by five adults. My mom was really dysfunctional, and I didn't realize that until I went to therapy. My uncles and my aunts, all of whom have since passed, were the stability in my life. The three guys were just incredibly funny and I always linked them to the Marx Brothers and Margaret Dumont, with my aunt being Margaret Dumont and my uncles being Harpo, Chico, and Groucho. It was fun. I could not think of a better way to grow up, even though it wasn't quite your average Ozzie and Harriet's '50s family. It was pretty amazing that my mother carried me to term in '53. It's an amazing fact that nobody in the neighborhood, or the church I belonged to, ever made a big deal about it.

Everybody was working, so we had a ton of dough coming through the house. Mom didn't go back to work until I was about eight. She was a histologist, my uncle was a manager, and one uncle had retired early. My aunt worked for the railroad company. There was tons of money going through the house. We were basic middle-class meat-and-potatoes people. We weren't driving Mercedes or stuff like that, but we were all comfortable. I don't remember anybody ever wanting anything. I went to a public grade school—a private Lutheran high school—and then to a state university.

My family was completely and totally unchurched—absolutely, totally unchurched. It was really a freewheeling kind of household. It was kind of "Try anything," which is how the faith came to me. The next-door neighbor said, "You know, send my daughter and Adam to summer school together." I remember my uncle was kind of the alpha dog in the family and he said, "Oh, it can't hurt." We got sent to the church.

I always loved organ music and the church had put in a brand new pipe organ. I was just astounded by watching them being able to build it and watching it, listening to the way it sounded. I'm stilled enthralled by pipe organs. If anything, God came really through the music, and still does, even though I'm the preacher. A great organist and the blast of a wonderful instrument and music are all important parts of what I do.

I don't remember my teenage years being terribly traumatic, but I do remember being unbelievably confused because I was clearly drawn not in the way that everybody else was. I remember having just this awful crush on the guy with whom I double-dated to prom. I still dated women. In those days, which were late '60s, that was expected. One went to the prom with women; one dated women. I was a moderate jock. I was a swimmer, not like the football player jock. I always was looking and had a terrible crush in the guy I went to prom with, even though he wasn't the person I went to prom with. Then I had a series of tumultuous crushes on guys but never acted on them.

What I do remember is, strangely enough, there was an awful lot of wrestling going on. I met a guy who was just finishing high school. He and I would just wrestle for hours and then do some very odd things. We would go running late at night and go skinny dipping in my backyard pool. Clearly, had I known then what I know now! I remember thinking back to, "What if we did something, tried something, and he got mad and the friendship would be over?" That was the clear fear—that I would lose him as a friend if I tried something. That was basically my case through high school and college.

I did tons and tons of things around the church. I was kind of a church rat. Sang in the choir and did youth group stuff, always Lutheran. That was pretty much the center of my social life.

I went on to seminary. It was a wonderful experience in that people used to say that it was the place to go if you were gay. I discovered we had this really attractive freshman class and a gay admissions director. That's where I discovered who I was. I could not have had a better coming out.

A friend of mine, who I thought was just gorgeous the minute I saw him, would come down in the morning to have coffee with me, and we did that for, like, 3 or 4 months. We sat together and we watched the *CBS Morning News* with Diane Sawyer and we would just have coffee. Then he told me he was gay. Then, in a magic 3-week period of time, we had a gay couple on campus come out to the church newspaper. They went to the church newspaper telling them they were gay, as opposed to going to their bishop. Well, they got thrown out of school. There was this big dustup and some controversy.

My friend would still come down and have coffee. Then we did the usual. He started by saying the famous line of every gay man, "Would you like a back rub?" We traded back rubs for a couple of nights.

Then I remember my existential crisis was that my primary uncle was a major hockey fan, and I was a fan since I was a little kid. I remember laying on the floor of my room in seminary with my giant head phones, listening to the hockey game thinking, "If I'm gay, will I still be a hockey fan?" I was buying in to all the stupid stereotypes.

About a couple of days after the couple was expelled from school, we had a week dedicated to sexuality. The last Friday evening, a guy at evening prayer preached about the 139 Psalm, which I can quote for you from memory: "Lord you have searched me and known me, my lying down and my rising up. If I ascend to the mountains you are there. If

I descend to the depths, you are there also. Such knowledge is too wonderful. Before I was knit together in my mother's womb you knew me."

The preacher said, "Whoever you are, God knew you and loved you before you were knit together in your mother's womb. You are fearfully and wonderfully made. Now go. Be about that business, the living that turns out to be for you."

I remember—this sounds sappy, like a bad movie—I was going to dinner at a friend's: the woman I was dating and the guy who ultimately brought me out. We're walking north and I said to myself, "Now who would you rather be with?" I went to dinner and the next morning my male friend and I did the deed for the first time. That was Saturday and the hockey game was on Saturday night, and I still loved the sport.

The most amazing thing was that the sun didn't come up in the west. Nothing was changed. And I wasn't, all of a sudden, flaky. Nothing was any different. Except that now I knew who I was and felt very good about it.

My mother and I were never close. We couldn't walk across the street without fighting. So, we never got along. She went to the grave with me never having the conversation, telling her that I was gay, because I figured she knew. She hated every woman that I ever brought home and she hated every guy that I ever brought home. So I figured she made the connection and there you go. But she was just a pistol; there was nothing I could do right in her eyes.

After the seminary, I picked a church—wonderful church, bad town. I had a great supervising pastor and the first thing he asked was: "What ear would you pierce if you want to tell people you are gay?"

I asked, "Why? Are you thinking of having your ear pierced?"

And he said, "No, but the guy who just left, in a premarital counsel, has his ear pierced." Then he and I had wonderful discussions about everything.

I really wanted to go back to Chicago because, I cannot tell you, even though I did meet somebody out there and we had a great time, if you didn't go and drink beer, you were pretty much out of the social scene. I used to say, "It didn't have none of the glories of a big city, none of the charms of a small town." It was this big industrial clump.

I was offered a job at a parish on the far North Side of Chicago by a pastor who I knew. I was with him for 6 years and that was probably the darkest period of my life. We also had talks about sexuality and that kind of thing. Somehow, I think because he became an alcoholic, he threatened to out me. This was back in the day when it was not permitted to be a gay Lutheran clergyman. He threatened to out me if I didn't find another job. He felt really threatened by my presence there. Needless to say, it ruined our the relationship and I found work. I quickly found another gig and left. It was probably the darkest time.

I learned about HIV when I was in the seminary. We had seminars on the topic. I'm kind of one of these guys who, if there is an interesting thing, I read everywhere about it. I kind of kept in front of it.

In a strange little aside: I have a congenital urinary stricture. One of the things is that, for me to be a top, if I get a urinary infection, it often closes up entirely and that means an emergency catheterization, which is not a pleasant experience. So I was wearing condoms before condoms were cool. The last thing I wanted was a urinary infection. Still, if there is one thing I'm afraid of is a urinary tract infection: Death through urinary tract infection.

The best friend of one of my roommates became sick and died of AIDS, when it began. We lost the admissions director to AIDS, due to complications. We never quite said that he died of AIDS; he died of pneumonia. Then I lost a couple more friends to it.

I am positive. Here is me, the big dumb oaf. I became positive 2 years ago. My therapist got me through beating myself up over making that stupid mistake. I'd say, "No, it was because I was stupid and did unprotected sex. I'm sure the guy didn't know. It takes two to be stupid."

I took it very well and take my meds every day. My doctor and I waited around for a year; my numbers were good for about a year, then they got a little higher than we wanted them to be. I have a great physician. He talks, he shares, he tells you everything you need to know and things you don't need to know. Then he said, "I think you probably should start taking medication for HIV." I started on Sustiva and had a horrendous reaction, so we stopped that immediately.

One Sunday morning I looked at my body in the mirror before I started my shower and I said, "Oh my God! I must be sick. I must be really sick." My body was covered in a discolored rash. I had to work. Fortunately, there was nothing on my face.

I called my friend up in a panic, and he said, "It's the meds. You have to stop the meds. It can't be anything else. People don't just turn funny colors."

The doc took me off of everything for a couple of months until my system cleared. I started up again and I've been fine ever since. What I want to tell people is, "Listen, you guys, I consider myself to be an incredibly lucky man. I haven't had any side effects, my life is not going to end, but I wouldn't wish this on my worst enemy."

My sexual life is back on and good. I don't play around as much as I did, with multiple partners. I have sex with friends who know and we play cheerfully. The hard part is telling your dentist and everybody on the list, and all of them saying, "Aren't you a little old for this kind of stuff?"

"Yeah let's not get into that. I'm really embarrassed."

Then there was a guy who I had a couple of coffee dates with. We had a couple of coffee dates, and I asked, "Would you like to see if we can stand each other to do dinner?" It was right after I had the rash thing, so I told him the funny story, which I thought was humorous, because I'm a good-humored guy.

He sent me a-n email that said, "That's a deal breaker for me and I can't have a relationship with you."

I was just flabbergasted by that, because that seems to me to be discriminatory. I wrote him back and I said, "Does this mean that dinner is off? There's no chance of a friendship with an HIV man?"

He wrote me back, "No, that's pretty much a deal breaker." I thought to myself it was tantamount to the "n" word. You just can't say, because of someone's status, "I'm not going to associate with you."

Fortunately, I went to therapy and talked about it. Of course, the therapist said the obvious thing, which I knew: that it was better to know then than to find out later that he was this way.

Now my basic personal life motto is: I only discriminate against people who discriminate. I was bothered by it. I was bothered by it more than I could think I was going to be bothered. I'm the WASP poster boy. There is no discrimination in my life; nobody discriminated me in my life. And because I can run under the radar as far as my sexuality goes, people who don't want to know, do not know about my sexuality. It was devastating. It was the first time for me.

In the gay scene, there is an unwritten discrimination. Geez, there are a lot of guys looking for daddies, but you can clearly see if you look at bars that the young guys are with the young guys and the older guys are with the older guys. There isn't a lot of interaction between them. Where I've seen that break down entirely is in places like gay resorts. The times I have stayed at gay resorts, late at night, over drinks in a hot tub, there are all kinds and conditions of people, of all ages, sitting there, sharing stories about what they did, where they went. People sitting there—absolutely stark raving naked—talking about the evening, without sex rearing its head. I find that to be just a glimpse of the Kingdom of God. I really do think it's the way it ought to be. We all talking to each other and not hitting on each other. And the older guys aren't hitting on the younger guys, which I find inappropriate, unless the younger guy comes on to me.

My personal trainer is in his late 20s, and when I tell stories about growing up, he looks at me like I'm a mammoth. He cannot believe them. "You really felt compelled to go to the prom with a woman?" he asked.

"Yes!"

He looked at me like I had suddenly become a dinosaur. There's a fascinating study to be made, to say, get an old guy with a young guy together and have them share stories, because it's just stunning.

I'm still a jock. I swim or lift weights 5, sometimes 6, days a week if I have enough time. I'm as healthy as a man can possibly be. I have an incredible drive. My doctor claims he is a vegetarian and I, like, eat garbage and my cholesterol is 100 points lower than his is. It's just good genes; it's friends, friends that I've met at the AGLO mass, which is run by the Archdiocesan Gay and Lesbian Organization.

My life is basically great. I'm, for the most part, happy in my job. I like my house. I love sitting out in the yard. I have a whole bunch of good gay and straight friends. Other people would look at the conditions and say, "Boy, you're positive, you're gay, you don't have a partner." But, I enjoy having ice cream with my buddies on Halsted Street, and sitting in the window and watching the world go by. A good meal, a good show—it doesn't get better than that. I really am working, still, on a relationship, a long-term relationship.

JESSE

"I Am a Chameleon; I Adapt to Whatever You Throw Me Into"

WHEN WE ARE OLDER, I think we are more mature. We have a lot more knowledge about life and experiences. At my age, I've done a lot of different things. I think I'm more mature than I was 20 years ago, but I don't consider myself as being old at 56. I'm older but not old.

I've been in Chicago a total of 30 years. I lived here for 25 years, then moved back to Indiana for 5 years to take care of my dad until he passed away. I was gone for 5 years, and since then I've been back. I was born in Ohio. I went to Indiana when I was 13 to live with my father and my stepmother, after being here in Chicago with my biological mother. I was a wild teenager; it was best that I went to live with my dad. That was the best thing that ever happened to me: to leave Chicago and to go live with my dad with five children and my stepmom, who was very grounded. It just couldn't have been a better choice for me at that time. I don't regret it.

I graduated from high school and went straight into the automobile industry. I worked there for 6 years until the oil–Japanese crisis, and then I got laid off. I went to Chicago to visit my mom and never left. I went to a school for computerized accounting, then I started working in a private corporation as a clerk, and worked my way up to credit and collections supervisor. I did that for 8 years. Then I went to a credit company, collecting guaranteed student loans. I did that for another 10 years. After I got tired of being on the phone, I went into decorating. I've been doing floral arrangements ever since, on my own.

I have a very close family. I have a daughter of 37 and two grandchildren. I was married for 4 years and got divorced. Me and my mother don't have a very good relationship. We are sort of estranged. I'm closer to my stepmother than I am to my mom. Me and my dad were very close in my later years versus my younger years. I'm very close with all of my siblings, nieces and nephews, my daughter, my grandchildren, and everybody seems to respect me and accept me. They all know I'm homosexual. They all knew my lover, who I was with for 15 years and had a beautiful relationship until the day that he passed away, unfortunately. He died in '95, of AIDS. We tested HIV positive in '86, together. After that, me and my family got along well. They all respect me and treat me like family.

When I came out at 28, I was in Chicago. My sister and I talked. My family expected me to wear a dress and have finger nails and wear wigs, and when they saw me walk in, it was the same me. I walked the same way! "The only difference about me is that I am in love with and I am living with a man now."

Being wasn't much of a surprise. I knew it, but I always fought it and never accepted it. I hid it and was ashamed of it until I came out. I came to Chicago and that's what made me feel comfortable, because I started seeing other people like me. There was nobody different than I, unlike in high school and elementary school, where everybody was straight. I had to be straight and act straight, have a baby and have a girlfriend, and do what I thought would make my dad proud. But nothing made him prouder than me being happy, and I'm a happy person. I don't regret my life at all. I know I've made some not-too-good decisions by becoming HIV positive, but it happened. I accept it and I've been very, very blessed.

As a child, we were not stable living with my mom. It was me, my mother, and my older brother. We moved from apartment to apartment, from school to school. It was just not a good, stable environment, because she was always doing something. I didn't have that "Donna Reed" and *Father Knows Best* life. I had a real rough childhood. I was living with a single mom who didn't have an education and lived the street life. Me and my brother were left alone: "Here's $5. Get yourselves something to eat and I'll see you all later."

I did not go to school like I was supposed to. I did what I wanted to do because I didn't have any guidance. That was my life with my mom. We don't see eye to eye on a lot of things. I disagree with the way she had five kids and gave up all but two of them. I don't have a lot of respect for my mother. I love her because she is my mother, but she could have been a better person. She doesn't feel like she's done anything wrong. Let's see, I have two sisters I don't know, I got a baby brother I have never seen.

With my older brother, the one I lived with, there were differences. I'm light skinned with supposedly good hair;

he's dark skinned with supposedly nappy hair. He's short; I'm tall. He used to whoop my butt all the time and call me "pussy" and that all that other crap.

We didn't have a stable home, but we always had a place to stay. I went to every elementary school in the area. Every one of them. But there is not one school that I finished the whole school year at, throughout my entire childhood, from kindergarten on up.

I am a chameleon. I adapt to whatever you throw me into. I'm a survivor. I got to do what I got to do to survive. I adapted. I adapted because I wanted to. I wanted to change. The only thing I regretted about moving to Indiana was the deception by my mother of me going there to visit my father for a week, then finding out, "No, we are going to enroll you in school. You're staying here. You're not going to Chicago." I felt like my mother gave me away like she did all her other kids. I had just turned 13.

Then I was in a family of six kids. I had a mother and a father. They had four children together and she had one prior to marrying my father, and then me. It was a mother and a dad, six kids; and I went to school. When I came home from school, there were four pots on the stove for dinner. You ate, you mopped the floor, you took out the garbage, and you did your homework. I was an A student. I went to school every day, I went to church every Sunday, had new clothes; I felt comfortable. I had friends who liked me, and cousins and aunts; it was a family. I loved it. I really did. I appreciated it so much. I think it made me a better person to grow up in that environment.

My stepmother is a firm believer in going to church every Sunday. We had to get up, go to school, and go to church. She is a firm believer in God, and a firm believer in doing the right thing and being good to other people.

When Martin Luther King was killed and they were doing all the riots, my Dad said, "You guys are lucky. You never had to experience prejudice." We were the first black family in an all-white neighborhood in Indiana, and we went to an all-white school, but didn't live in the all-black neighborhoods, which were right around the corner, but separated. There was an imaginary fence. We just didn't have any racial tension or prejudice, that people called you "nigger" or anything like that. I never experienced it.

I graduated from high school and went to university. I wanted to be an accountant. I liked numbers and I was good in math. But that was my aspiration. I didn't finish school because I had a child in high school and got married. I had to work, take care of my wife, and take care of my daughter. We were boyfriend and girlfriend from eighth grade on and we had a child in our senior year of high school. After 4 years, I couldn't stand her and she couldn't stand me. I left her the house and got my own place; we got a divorced and went our separate ways. But, to this day, we love each other. I'm a good dad, at least my daughter tells me so. I've always been a good dad. When my daughter was 13, I told her I was gay. I was living with a man in Chicago and she was still living in Indiana with her mom. She said, "You'll always be my dad." From that point on, I could care less what someone else thought of me.

When I moved to Chicago, I was on the North Side, and one day I walked down Oak Street. I went into this bar, a gay bar, but I didn't know it was a gay bar. Guess who was sitting in the gay bar? My cousin!

He said, "What you doing here?"

I said, "I just moved here."

He started introducing me to his friends.

I asked, "Is this a gay bar?"

He said, "Yup."

For some reason, I just felt comfortable. I've been called "sissy" all my life, have a high-pitched voice, and don't play sports. I always played with girls when I was living with my mom; never did anything with any guys—always with my girl cousins, female friends, and my mother's friends. My uncles used to call me a sissy, my older cousin used to call me a sissy, and they pushed me aside. When I moved to Chicago at 10, I was with my cousin on the South Side and you didn't play with girls. That made me tougher and made me come out more as a boy, because I was around a lot more boys. We did a lot of bad things: stayed out all night, smoked reefer, smoked cigarettes, drank wine at 12 years old, didn't go to school. That was my life during that period.

When I moved to Indiana after that, I was around my two younger brothers, my older stepbrother, older cousin, and my dad. I just didn't want to be that sissy anymore. I wanted to be a boy. I wanted to be a man. And I was a man, even to this day. I never had anyone in Indiana, or at any job that I've had in my adult life, disrespect me.

I experimented with my stepbrother and my cousin. I didn't really have a sexual experience until I was 25 years old, after I got divorced. That's when I knew that I was gay. That's when I knew that out of all those years that I really did have some type of attraction to another man.

When I moved to Chicago, I went to the bathhouses. I met my lover in a bathhouse—that one night—and we were together for 15 years.

People were dying. I guess AIDS was more in New York and in San Francisco. It didn't affect our immediate friends. AIDS was seen more with white men than black men. So, it didn't occur to us that we might be infected, or get infected. But then, when our closer friends became infected, we decided to get tested. That's when my lover and I found out that, in all of our rambunctiousness, we had been exposed to the virus. My cousin died (the one I met at the bar) from AIDS. A lot of our friends passed away from AIDS. My lover withered before my eyes, just like a leaf on a tree. I saw him lose his hearing, lose his eye sight, and wither away like a leaf. I took care of him until I took him back to Detroit to his mom. My lover was African American and 5 years older than me.

I think one of the reasons why I'm still here today is because, when I was watching my lover, I never took those pills that were given back then. I didn't take anything until after his death, in '95.

At that point, my doctor told me, "You better start doing something. You got 5 years to live."

That's when I started a regimen. But I would be so sick and so exhausted with diarrhea and fatigue that I would take the medication for 6 months and then stop it for a year.

The doctor said, "You are going to have to take it all the time."

I always felt better without the medicine than I did taking the medicine. I went to work and I kept my job. I didn't feel any need to take the meds. I believe now that some people died from the medicine. I believe they died more from taking the AZT than they did from the actual virus.

Five or 4 years ago, I told my doctor, "I'm through taking the four pills in the morning and the six pills at night—the diarrhea and the fatigue; I'm just tired of it."

He said, "They just came out with this new pill. You only take one pill a day."

"Okay," I said, "Let's give that a try." My viral load and my T-cell count have just been perfect for me; no fatigue, no diarrhea. I have been undetectable for 5 years and my T cells were 300 last time I checked.

HIV was a death sentence back then. But my resolve was that I wasn't sick, I didn't get sick. I didn't buy in to all the hoopla that because you are HIV, you're going to die tomorrow. I didn't feel that way and I was healthy. My doctor said I was healthy. I didn't have any signs. I wasn't in the hospital, like I was seeing my friends who would die rapidly. I didn't experience any of that. I was going to work when my lover was at home.

The same way I told my family I was gay, I said, "We tested and I'm HIV positive." My stepmother, who is very religious, was very afraid for me. But what she did, that I thought was miraculous for her being in the Stone Age, was that she read up on it and educated herself to where we could talk about it.

My mother, my biological mother in Chicago, was a nurse assistant and she knew. She'd seen it with her own eyes because a lot of guys on her floor died. She was in that AIDS ward.

Another reason why we don't get a long is because I found out I had three insurance policies for over a million dollars in my name that I knew nothing about. My mother took them out with a friend of hers who had an insurance scheme going. They took these three policies out in the span of 9 years and I knew nothing about it. So I ended up testifying against her and against him. Me and my stepmother wanted to kill my mother, "Why were you banking on me to die?"

I think it's my attitude that has helped me. It's my attitude, my belief in myself, and not letting anyone else bring me down, because I have too much to live for, I have too many people that love me that I love, and I love my life. I really, really do. I'm very secluded, I'm very private, and I don't weigh down my problems on everybody. I walk around feeling like I'm very, very blessed. I feel good about being here and being able to live. I have beautiful grandchildren. Me and my daughter are very close—very, very close—and that's such a special relationship. Me and my stepmother have a beautiful relationship. The last 5 years I took care of my dad, we had a beautiful relationship. He had never once said anything to me about being gay. Never. Nothing negative came out of his mouth. We talked about everything in the world, but me being gay. He treated my partner like he treated any other friend of mine. I will go to my death believing two things: that my dad respected me enough not to degrade me about my homosexuality, and that me and my lover had a monogamous relationship.

I think I'm so strong because of my childhood. When you live such a hard or deprived life, or when you have to really, really fight at 8 years old to survive, by yourself, it's easy when you are 28 to get a job and an income. I got my self-esteem, I have my pride, and I bank on it. I think that's what keeps me sustained.

My best friend likes fur coats and going to the bar; this is all funny to me. I do all of his taxes and pay all his bills on the computer, because he doesn't know nothing about computers! He likes depending on me for things like that, and I like being around because we laugh and talk, and we love each other, and we've been friends for 25 years. We depend on one another and we never had a sexual inclination toward one another. He's my longest friend today who's alive. I had a lot of friends—. We just got together Tuesday night last week. A friend of ours from California was here. I hadn't seen those people in over a year, because I hadn't been to the bar, the Second Story.

I said, "There's one thing about not seeing you—I don't have to see you every day, I don't have to talk to you on the phone every day—but when I'm able to see you, we pick up right where we left off, as though we were together yesterday."

This little young guy, who is HIV positive, and me have sex once or twice a month. I can go months without any sex. It doesn't bother me. I don't have to have sex every day. When I do have sex, I enjoy it. I'm on it. But I'm just not like him. He's 33 and wakes up every single day: "Oh, I got to have sex. I got to have it."

No you don't. You think you do, but you don't have to. Even with my partner, we were together for 15 years; we didn't have sex every day. I still have a good erection, I still enjoy sex; it's a nice part of life, but it is not my life. Me and that younger guy were lovers for 6 years after my lover died. That young guy wanted sex every day and we did it every day. That's what broke us up. I could not do it every day.

"Being a top and you being a bottom—I'm sorry, but I just don't function like that." It turns me off to be aggressive in that manner. It got to the point where I didn't mind—you go, go to the bathhouse.

I'm very afraid of sexual diseases, very afraid of catching syphilis, Chlamydia, or gonorrhea. I had syphilis before and I didn't know what to do. It was detected immediately and I got taken care of immediately. I'm really afraid of catching diseases, so I don't like being promiscuous. I'm not a promiscuous type of guy. I like one person and I like being able to depend on that person. That's my idea of sex. I love passion and intimacy; I think it's the most important part of sex. If I just want to jack off, then I can do that. I really enjoy being intimate and feeling the passion. That's the best part of sex—the passion and the longevity. And I haven't been to a bathhouse in 10 years.

I don't feel old and I don't carry myself—. Well, I'm not no hip-hopper like these young kids, but I'm comfortable with my life. My friends and I do a lot of potlucks; we do a lot of house gatherings with our immediate friends, over at my friends' or my house. We listen to music and eat—mostly eat and drink. It's either somebody's birthday, Thanksgiving, or Christmas, or we just get together to watch a basketball game or a football game. One friend loves sports and another loves to cook; add a big TV screen and it's a party. I like doing things because I don't do them every day. I'm a homebody. I love to read and write. I read murder mysteries. I'm a little aggressive in the political arena and very in tune to what's happening politically. I watch all the political shows and news.

If I'm out and I'm attracted to someone, they do say, "Oh, you're too old for me." Because they don't think I can keep it up or last long. Then, when I tell them that I'm on Social Security and not working, and don't have a Mercedes in the driveway—I'm not a sugar daddy—they look at that.

If you're older, the younger guys think you're supposed to have money and be able to take care of them. "I'm not taking care of no kids!" I got a granddaughter who's graduating from high school next year. I'm trying to get an airplane ticket so I can go see her, and then she's got college to go to. That's what I'm looking forward to! "I'm not looking to take care of you!" That's where my money is going to: my granddaughter.

I got an 8-year-old grandchild, and I'm looking forward to him going to high school in 3 years. So I don't got time for somebody else's kids. I want somebody who can take care of himself. And I say, I shouldn't, but I don't think I'll ever find anybody like my deceased lover. Really, my first lover—I don't think I'll ever have that relationship again.

I'm retired now. I live by myself, got a nice studio apartment on the South Side. Been there 3 years. I'm most satisfied with me being not a burden to anybody else. I'm independent; I can take care of myself. I'm loved and respected by my friends and my family. I really don't have any problems that I can't take care of. I'm not going to say that I have a perfect life, because I don't, but I'm pretty happy with myself. I have an 86-year-old aunt, who I think I spend too much time with, but I love her, and she depends on me and I like doing things for her. We go out to dinner, and go to Walmart and walk around there for hours. I spend a lot of my time doing things like that, or I spend a lot of time alone, and it doesn't bother me.

I wish I had more money, but I can pay my bills. I don't owe anybody. I detest borrowing money. Things are expensive, but I think I do damn well. I'm not needy for anything. I'm not homeless, I got a nice wardrobe, I can look nice for any occasion. I can go anywhere, do anything, and you don't know I don't got a job because I don't look like I don't have one. So I fit in. I'm a chameleon! The only thing I'm pissed off about is that I've been 160 lb and 32 waist size since the 12th grade. Now I'm 188 lb and waist side 36 in 2 years, and I am pissed. I am pissed! I don't like that man in the mirror.

My immediate plan is to make sure that my granddaughter graduates from high school next year and that she goes to college. I see her through college and I see her becoming the pharmacist that she wants to become. That's my immediate plan. And my grandson, also. As for me, I don't have any plans for me. I'm just living, taking it day by day. As long as I don't have anything major to come down to disrupt my life, I think I can make it. If I'm needed, I want to be there for the people who need me. I don't have any money, but I can do something.

LOUIS

"I'm Always Meeting the Underdog People"

I HAVE BEEN IN CHICAGO all my life. I'm 54, going to be 55 next month. I've lived all over Chicago: south, west, north, southwest, and east. I live alone. I've been a year by myself now. I love it. I guess I'm retired. I was working in a nursing home. I was a floor technician. I got the HIV virus right in '99 and was assigned light duties.

The case manager said to me, "Why don't you quit and get disability?"

I said, "No. I don't want to. I want to work."

But that was in 1999, when there were a lot of things opening up for HIV people. That was an opportunity I passed on because I liked working. But then I got sicker and stopped working. I got disability, so that's what made me stop working. I'm not looking to be rich and famous, but I'm comfortable by myself. I paint and listen to music 24/7. I love jazz, contemporary jazz, because it's my music, and I love animals.

I used to be a male hustler. Then I got a good job at McDonald's headquarters in Oakbrook. I was a mail clerk there and I had to quit that place, too, and I started being a male hustler again. I said, "Well, I'm not a bank robber. I'm not a murderer. I'm not a stick-up person," so I went to Social Security and applied for disability and they denied me. I got a public lawyer. She was very nice; I'll never forget her. She looked at my case and I got on disability for a learning disability.

I have no boyfriend. I have best friends. I have three best friends that I've known for 30 or 40 years now. They are male and they are gay. They've been with me through more than what I've been with them! But as far as a companion, I don't have one. I would like to have one, but it's nothing that I'm looking or shopping for. I do go out and dance a lot because I like dancing.

I'm on a fixed income, so I don't have time to baby-sit anyone or try to take care of anyone. And most of the people I've met, they have drug issues, like I used to have. I used to be a drug addict. I'm still in recovery.

For some reason, I'm always meeting the underdog people. I used to do that a lot, which was one of my downfalls in life. I used to pick up the underdog and they never knew what issues I was going through. I never shared. I would like a relationship. I think I'm ready for one now, but it just has to happen.

I had a good childhood, or so I think it was good to me. I remember, in kindergarten, skipping school. I had about six to seven dogs, alley dogs that I would play with. I would hide in this abandoned garage on the West Side during the school day and I would feed them and play with them. Then, I'd hear the bell ring and I would put them in the garage, close the door, and go back to school like I'd been there all day. That went on for, like, 3 or 4 months, until the truant office called my mother. They told my mother I had not been in school for, like, 2 months. I got busted. In kindergarten, I wasn't a good reader or anything, but just felt I was more advanced than my classmates. The coloring and whatever didn't interest me. Nature and animals are what interested me when I was that age.

I remember having a good life. I was the youngest. I really didn't have that much parental guidance. I was a day dreamer. My mother and father were around, but they were always working or my mother was going to play bingo. My older brothers and sisters were doing their thing. They really didn't want to be bothered with me. So I made my own world, I guess. And I was happy with it.

My father worked for the post office and my mother was a nurse. There were four of us at that time and then my mother got remarried in 1968, and she had three others. So there's three older than me and three younger than me. I was in the middle. My mother and father are still alive. I loved my stepfather, because he actually was the one who taught me how to tell time. They didn't have digital clocks then.

My mother would argue, "This child doesn't know how to tell time!"

He said to me, "When you learn, I'll buy you your first watch."

I respected that about him. He was a good stepfather. He really was. He was more a father to me than my actual father was, at the time. My stepfather has passed, but my real father is still alive. I get along with him. He still could whoop us but he's in his late 70s; he's cool. My mom is still vibrant. She lives in Michigan, still doing her thing, not letting any of her kids stand in her way. I have a lot of her traits, I think.

Teenage years were the bizarre years. But it was good, too; it was really good. I had a good teenager life. I started having sex early, really early—at 10. I started having a lot of girlfriends because I liked sex and I liked girls. I always fantasized about the perfect wife and the picket fence and kids. I always knew I wanted to have kids. But then I didn't know about my sexuality.

In my teenager life, I did a lot of plays in high school: *West Side Story, Death of a Salesman*, and *Guys and Dolls*. That's when I got exposed to different cultures and people with different sexualities.

I grew up in the projects, so I was like the leader because most of my peers couldn't do as much as me because their mothers where at home 24/7. My mother was not. They always came to me about how to talk to girls. I would say, "Be yourself, have a good sense of humor, and don't lie."

Then, at like 16 or 17, I started meeting guys in summer school. I started having that notion more and more, but I fought it because my girlfriend at that time got pregnant. Then I got another girl pregnant the same year. A boy was liking me in summer school and he was very handsome. I will never forget his name and how he looked. He was very handsome. We had a little conversation and so forth.

I didn't know if I liked boys or girls. I just knew I liked the sex a lot—a lot! It was a good teenager life. It really was. There were my mother, my grandmother, and my aunt; there were no uncles. So we were raised basically by a bunch of strong black women who believed in education, mannerisms, clear speaking, and good habits. That was all getting in my head.

I wanted to be myself. I wanted to try to be a hippie. But things started getting rough really after the kids began being born. I knew I liked the boys and I knew I liked the girls; it was getting complicated. I still think about those days. I really had good people in my life. I could have gone a whole other route, like a lot of my peers back then—in jail for rape, murder, stuff like that.

I stopped going to high school. My mother was at work and she didn't know. I started having parties with girls at the house. I was the only one who was home at that time. I was, more or less, basically on my own. There was no supervision. As I said earlier, I had three siblings, younger siblings. My mother and her mother used to always get into a fight about her leaving the kids with me because I was, like, 12 years old, but I didn't mind. After I would feed them, my mother would go to work and then she'd go to bingo. She'd sleep; she'd leave. I would play with the kids, wear them out, and they would go to sleep. Then I would go out. That's when I got introduced to a gay environment.

I went to one gay bar when I was in my early 20s. I didn't like it because I thought I would start to be a drag queen—that's what type of bar it was. "Maybe that's what would happen to me." I didn't like their style, but to each his own. I didn't go out anymore until another friend of mine introduced me to these underground clubs, for the people with a normal life like me. That's when I said, "OK. Now I'm ready."

But I actually wasn't ready until my youngest daughter was born. (She's 24 or 25 now.) I stopped and got married. I tried to do the right thing. Then I was doing drugs: acid, speed, this and that. I wanted to get married because she was a good woman and my first kid's mother, so I did. That was a struggle, because we were in the projects for 19 years.

We had a good sex life and plus I knew her from special ed in high school.

After my youngest daughter was born, I had a boyfriend, too. I couldn't tell my wife, even though she asked about my gayness because she went out to the underground clubs with me, and there were a lot of gay people there, too. She would ask and I would deny it, because at that time I had no job, no income, so I had to have insurance, really, and somewhere to live. That's really what I was looking at. I didn't want to live with my siblings. I didn't want to live with my mother anymore. After my youngest daughter was born, then I did come clean and tell my wife. She was upset, but she didn't get hysterical like some women do; she would never get that hysterical.

So, I said, "I got to go. I got to go somewhere. If it was in the street, I would have to do that."

Then she would say, "No, you don't have to leave."

It was getting hard. Times were changing and life was going by so fucking fast. I realized my luck was starting to fade.

My feelings toward men, actually started when I was younger and I just didn't see it. I wasn't a butchie and my friends weren't butch. I always knew—when I'd see men, they looked handsome. I always noticed that and admired that. Maybe I repressed it a lot as I got older. I still knew men were handsome looking, but I was not as much as physically attracted to them. But the handsome part, it turned me on.

After I separated, then I'd go with males always. I moved out and I was still with males, but a lot of females were attracted to me. I had problems really going to bed with another female because I wouldn't even get an erection. I liked their beauty, but not the sex part. Women liked my gentlemanhood. I'm attracted to men, so I never acted bisexual. I never thought I was bisexual. I always knew I was just gay. I never could let it go because of the circumstances.

I started smoking weed early, and then when I started going to underground clubs, like at 17 or 18, I took acid. It progressed as I got older. I liked the feeling; I felt hippie. I felt more free to talk to other males or females. The drugs helped me blend in so well, that I could express to others how I really felt. It enhanced my feelings of talking about life and how sad I was. It progressed and progressed even more.

Nowadays, what's happening is the cancer thing. It's only been a year since I've had it. It's sort of spooky. The HIV wasn't spooky at all. But I got sick a lot of times with the HIV, until I started taking my medicines religiously. I went to the hospital several times for not taking medicines for the HIV. I'd get very, very sick—close to death.

My sister is a nurse and works in the cancer unit, so I have good family support. She's good, even though she's sort of a control freak like all the women in my family. It's OK. I'm used to it. We don't clash as much anymore because she's old and she helps. But I take my medicine religiously now and my HIV has been undetected for 3½ years.

The cancer came when I was in drug rehab. I had this great pain on both sides—on one side but then it progressed onto the other side. I went see my primary doctor for the HIV and I said, "Tell me what it is."

She said, "Well, I think it may be cancer."

When I found out, I was—still am—scared. Some days it's hard to swallow. Now I'm doing radiation. Even though my liver cancer is in remission, I have to take the chemo pills. I don't know; cancer gets sort of spooky to me at times. HIV is controllable if you take some pills, basically. But cancer, you don't know when—. I've been on the chemo pills since August of last year. They took me off them because I had bad side effects. Then I learned that cancer cells move around and now they think it's in my ribs and my lungs. That's why I'm doing the radiation now. I'm in a lot of pain in my ribs and my groin. Whether or not the radiation is killing the cells, I'm not sure. But cancer likely can just go overnight, move around, or you wake up the next day sick and in excruciating pain. What's good is that I have a good doctor; I appreciate my doctor. I'm very blessed.

I used to do the homecare for a man with HIV. He had AIDS, rather. He lived with his mother and father—strong black family, I thought. They were good to him. I would run errands and care for him at home. One day, I had to go to the hospital with him and he passed of AIDS. I wasn't scared, but I had to call his parents. I wasn't scared of HIV, but I told the agency, because they called me for another client. "No, I don't think I want this job." I couldn't deal with the depression of taking care of somebody dying. I connect with people somewhat too fast and believe in miracles. That's how I started finding out about HIV.

When I used to shoot up drugs, with a needle, I lived in the projects with my wife and kids. I used to shoot up with these two ladies. I didn't know how to do it myself. I didn't want to learn. One of these ladies died of AIDS. At that time, I wasn't really messing around with men as far as anal sex. I knew I got it from her—from sharing the needles. I did tell everybody, when I first found out. They didn't care, and that was 1999! So it's cool.

I'm the best cooker in the family—the one who cooks a barbecue. On certain occasions, I wear gloves when I cook, when we have family gathered, just to make myself comfortable too. But the family just asks how I feel some days. Then, on top of that, with the cancer, they've been a little bit overprotective than they were with the HIV.

I started dating this white guy who was really nice. He was in Michigan. I was working at a restaurant up north; he was working for the railroad. He was younger than me, but had a good job. He talked me into moving to Michigan, bought me a car, got me a job at the Federal Center, and got me my own apartment. He didn't live there, but lived somewhere else. I got nervous and decided to move back to Chicago, because his father was a policeman, and there I lived in an all-white community. He never let me meet any black people. I would tell him, "I'm not prejudiced. You know that. But I have to get some soul up in here. Where are the black men? Don't they have gay black men here?"

Yeah, I dated a few white men, and I still do on occasion. Sometimes I feel I have to prove to a white person that I'm intelligent. I'm just going to stand my ground because I love being a black African American. I think growing up I did have an identity crisis, because I was so dark and everybody else was light skinned. Back then, light people liked the dark people; dark-skinned people liked the light-skinned people. But that wasn't me. I always wanted to be with a dark man, but I was always getting chosen by light-skinned people. In those days, no dark-skinned person wanted a dark-skinned person. That was ludicrous to me. I can still see some light-skinned African Americans think they are superior to us dark-skinned black people.

I never had a problem with being gay after I realized that I was gay. But now it seems like a lot of people don't believe that I am, from my mannerisms. "What? Do I have to put on a dress or something? I'm gay! I need a boyfriend!"

It was never my thing to hang out with gay people. I never clicked. I'm going with the flow, actually, but I don't hide my gayness. I think African Americans, and hard core in the ghetto, sometimes if they see a gay person, and the person carries himself well, they have no problem; the straights respect him. They say, "OK, we got a faggot in the neighborhood." But ain't nobody going to mess with him, because he doesn't mess with anybody.

What helps me now go through life is seeing other people worse off than me. That makes me feel so blessed. It helps me be very kind to others. I go to an NA (Narcotic Anonymous) group on Fridays, I go to the Howard Brown (an older LGBT group), and then I got this new HIV group on Wednesdays. What I find is, in these groups, is that you never stop learning. Even though they say the same thing over and over at NA and HIV groups, somebody is going to say something I haven't heard, or somebody is going to be sitting in a pity pot and I want to try to cheer them up: "Get your ass off that pity pot."

I still think a whole lot about having sex. That's what I think about. Until I get some, I think about sex every 5, every 2 minutes. I'm always constantly thinking about sex. My closest friend calls me a "nympho." I want to meet somebody my age before we start dropping too much, so we can grow into love with each other. I'm scared. I don't want a young boy who has to go free someday. I want to be with somebody who's my age—maybe a couple of years younger—and we would grow older together.

It feels depressing, a little bit, but it feels good to have a life, because I thought I would be dead. When you get older, you get respect from people. I feel blessed; I really do. I feel so blessed. All my siblings are alive, and my mother and father. None of us is in jail or prison. All my kids are alive, my grandbaby. I feel good about my life. I just get lonely for a companion, but I deal with that by painting. But, you can only paint so much. Then I get so horny thinking about sex, but I can still see flowers and greenery.

The only thing I don't like about my life is that I got no hair and I'm getting a ball on my head! Yeah, I'm getting a ball. I don't like that. I wish I had hair or dreadlocks, so that at least I could do life with such hair. I thought the ball was fluid. The cancer people told me, "No, that's fat. Get on the treadmill." I go swimming. I love swimming.

I'm looking forward from day to day. I never was a planner for the future. I'm looking for another blissful day. I'm glad to get up in the morning and say, "OK, now what's the day going to bring to me?" Then I go to have my quiet moment for 45 minutes in the house with nothing on—TV, no music. Then I say, "OK, now you're ready." I try to put myself in a calm space because it's cruel out there; people can take you there. I just hope that I can stay in the calm place that I am.

JIMMY

"The Party Came to a Crashing End"

I AM 71. I WENT TO LAW SCHOOL. I was a lawyer before I retired. I was born in a farmhouse. It was 1939 and, during the Depression, my parents couldn't afford to take my mother to the hospital, so I was born at home. I have one brother and two sisters. They are all alive. My older sister is extremely ill; she's not expected to live much longer. After law school I moved to Chicago 1965.

There is some benefit of being older: you have a lot of first-hand experiences that young people don't have. They might hear about, "Well, you should do this; you should do that," but until you've actually done those things or gone through things that people go through, I don't think you really know as much about the world, yourself, and other people. I think growing old in that sense is an advantage. I try to keep myself physically active, so I don't really feel physically impaired at my age, although there are some things that you just can't do as well as you could when you were younger, like balance and that sort of thing. But I still am physically active as much as I can be. In fact, since I retired, a lot of my life has been about exercising. I bike 16 miles every other day during the summer months, the spring, and autumn, when the weather is nice. I do it outside around the lake. In the winter, I have a recumbent bike that I use at home.

Being a gay male in a big city like this, you don't get as much attention when you're older as you did when you were younger, but I don't know if that's a plus or a minus, actually. As far as growing older, I have changed my life. When I was younger, I would go to bars, I'd party more than I do now—or more than I have in the last 20 or 25 years. When you're younger, that sort of thing seems a lot more important than it does at the present time, at least for me.

Living on a farm, that was a big part of my life. I first became aware of the world during World War II. It seemed to be a scary time, because the young men were fighting against Japan, and they were fighting against Germany and Italy in Europe. Those memories are the most I think about when I think about being a child. We had air raid rehearsals, where you had to darken your house and you couldn't have any lights on. In retrospect, it seems kind of fanciful, because I don't think either Japan or Germany had the planes that could have gone all the way to the American Midwest. I suppose they didn't know that at the time.

I remember the day they said Hitler was dead. It was my birthday, my sixth birthday, 1945. I remember Roosevelt dying. I remember when the war completely ended in August, when Japan gave up, and hearing about the bombs, Hiroshima and Nagasaki. As far as my childhood is concerned, that was it.

I was jealous of my older sister and my brother because they went to school when I was still pretty young. I wanted to go with them, but I couldn't. I had to stay home with my mother and my little sister.

My father was a tenant farmer. We lived on a farm that was owned by his aunt. The tenant farmer got one half of the profit and the landlady, my great aunt, she got the other half. Farm boys were expected, in those days, to start helping work at a very young age. When I was maybe eight or nine, my father would get my brother and me up at dawn practically. We had to go out and feed the cattle and the hogs before we ate breakfast and before we went to school. In retrospect, I believe that was good. We didn't question it. We didn't talk back to our father and say, "Well, we don't want to do that." We just did it because we had to.

My parents took us to the local Baptist church, I believe, because that's where the neighbors went. The Baptist church in those days (I suppose today is still the same) professed to be very strict about a lot of things: drinking, dancing, fornicating, and premarital sex. Nobody said much about homosexuality back in those days, as if it didn't exist. Oh, and card playing was considered to be sinful by some of them. Most of it was hypocrisy, because the same people who claimed that all these things were awful, especially when it came to sex, were in fact not doing as they said.

When I became a teenager I came to a point where I dismissed religion as useless. Ever since, I have not been religious. I believe I might have been about 13 or 14 years old. One Easter Sunday, my parents were getting ready to go to church. It was a beautiful Easter Sunday and I liked to work in the vegetable garden. I told my mother and father that I was not going to go to church that day. I was going to stay home and I would spend my time with God that day in the garden and not in the church with the hypocrites. They didn't like it, but that's what happened.

When I was a teenager, the main thing, actually, was realizing that I was gay. I didn't necessarily accept it, but I had boyfriends, who were more than just friends. Most of what we did was mutual masturbation, although there were some of them I would go down on, but it never went beyond that. My first friend was when I was 11 years old—very close friends and we engaged in that sort of thing.

As a teenager, I came to realize that I liked to be with older people, rather than people my own age. I liked to talk about politics; I liked to read the newspaper, magazines, and books; and keep up on things and learn. I realized that I was going to be a bookish-type person. A lot of my contemporaries didn't want to think about those things; they wanted to think about childish things. So a lot of times, in social gatherings, I'd end up with the adults and I just talked with them.

It struck me as odd that I was supposed to find girls attractive. I did find them physically attractive, but I was supposed to have an attraction to them. I tried to develop it, and in fact I did have sexual relations with girls my own age when I was younger, even in law school I was still attempting to do it. I could do it, I could perform, but I was always thinking about guys; I was not thinking about the females.

It became clear, when I was about 15 or 16, that my desire for males was just a great deal more powerful than my desire for females. Nevertheless, this was back in the '50s and early '60s, when I was in law school, so in those days it wasn't terribly easy to admit to one's self, let alone the rest of the world, that you were queer or a faggot or anything like that. It just kept growing as the years went by, and by the time I graduated from law school, there was no hope for me anymore about being straight. By then I had given up all ideas of being straight. In fact, I sort of welcomed it.

I never liked the idea of being a father. I didn't think I would make a good parent, and I'm quite certain, in retrospect that, I wouldn't. It wouldn't have been a good idea for me to have been a father and it was sort of like, "Well, if you are gay, you don't have to do that." Although, now, a lot of gay and lesbians do raise children, and more power to them. I think that many times they are probably better parents than straight people.

I wasn't terribly successful finding guys in college and law school. I always had a friend, not all the way through law school, and there was mostly one person in college. Well, there was more than one in college, but there was a main person. He was my boyfriend; it was like *Brokeback Mountain*. The guys in one scene in *Brokeback Mountain*, one says, "I ain't gay," and the other guy says, "Neither am I." I don't think they say *gay*, I think they say *queer* or *faggot*, something like that. That was pretty much the way it was with my friend. We would beat off together, sometimes we'd kiss, and sometimes I would go down on him. Except, by the time I got to law school, I was saying, "I'm gay."

Then, when I went to Chicago after law school, I started working for one of the biggest law firms in the city. I found a person I had gone to college with there. I thought in college he was the queerest thing. I didn't have sexual relations with him, but he was so clearly gay. He introduced me to the bar scene in Chicago. I went to the bars, I met some guys, and that was it. I just took it from there. It was 1965.

I can't really recall anything negative about being in a same-sex relationship, other than the fact that I knew what society thought of people who were. If you were gay in those days, it was like you were a child molester or you were on a level of a serial murderer, in some people's minds. The best thing in my life, to be very frank, is the acceptance of gay people, because back in those days, you didn't even want to admit it to yourself. It was such a hellish thing to be and to do.

When I went to Chicago, I had some extremely unpleasant things happen because I'm gay. In the fall of 1966, I was still working for the big prestigious law firm, but two things happened. One was the Thanksgiving weekend of 1966. I went to a gay bar and there were some straight young men outside who were harassing the people who came and left. When I left the place with my boyfriend, we were both quite intoxicated. These young thugs followed us down the street yelling at us "faggots," "queer." I very stupidly told them to fuck off. There were more of them than I thought there were. They had knives and they cut me. They cut my face. There is a very light scar still in my forehead. I was covered with blood and I don't remember whether they thought they had killed me or not. I could have died, I suppose. I was a bloody mess.

At the same time, the people I worked with at the law firm, who considered themselves to be very liberal, found out I was gay. Another guy my same age worked there and we ran across each other in a gay bar one night. After that, he knew I was gay; I knew he was gay. He was joking around with other young lawyers and he told them that I knew where all the gay bars in Chicago were. I said, "Yeah, and you know where they are too, because that's where you go." We were both dismissed. He was fired immediately and they forced me out. I was definitely fired for being gay. I was shocked that these people, who claimed to be so liberal, were not ready for gay people. They couldn't put up with having gay and lesbians in their law firm. I ran into any number of lawyers who worked for big law firms in Chicago; they were just as closeted as they could be, because they knew that if they let it be known that they were gay, they weren't going to stay there.

After that, I went to work for a legal aid agency. We did legal work for indigent persons. I did that from the beginning of '67 until '95. Then I went to work for the Cook County Public Guardian, and that's where I ended my career in 2001, when I retired.

I went through those things and they were bad, but they didn't stop me. I went on with my life. After being fired from that law firm, I realized I would never make the kind of money that lawyers made working for big prestigious law firms, and I didn't want to work for a smaller law firm. Therefore, I was a public service lawyer by default. I never told the people I worked with that I was gay. As the years went by, it became more obvious that I was. The people I worked with accepted it, because they truly were liberal. If I had stayed with that big law firm, I would have had to work 80 hours a week and go through that stuff that, really, in retrospect, I didn't want any part of anyway. I put in a decent 40-hour work week and I had plenty of time to enjoy life.

Enjoying life in those days was taking a trip with a friend to San Francisco or New York, which were, in those days, more advanced for gay people. You didn't have to worry so much about a bar being raided, especially after Stonewall. San Francisco was, in fact, viewed by a lot of my contemporaries here in Chicago as a Mecca. But I didn't want to get that far away from my family and, being a lawyer, you had to take the bar exam again in California, and I didn't see myself doing that. I remained in Chicago and I'm glad I did because it left me near my family.

When AIDS first came out, several friends of mine came down with a mysterious illness—several of them at the same time. I believe it was in '81 when the first of them died. They would suddenly get sick and then they would die. Several of my friends died that way. First people said, "Oh, it was the drugs." Gay men were taking drugs and so was I—acid and that sort of thing. I did drugs a lot with my contemporaries—of course, smoked pot. But at first, everybody was trying to say it was the drugs. Some people even tried to say it was the poppers [alkyl nitrites]. Then, later on, it was determined that it was a retrovirus.

I'm personally affected by it. I had had sexual relations with several of the people who died. I had one special boyfriend who I lived with, but I also had two other boyfriends, and we all lived together; it was a free-for-all. We were having sex and doing drugs with other men.

The two first houses I lived in during the late '60s, and all three during the '70s were party houses. I was a party person and the people I lived with were all party people. So, we came to the conclusion that we probably had the disease and we were probably eventually going to die. That was my feeling in the early '80s. It was like the party came to an end. It started in the late '60s and it went all the way through the '70s; but then in '80s, people (in their wisdom) elected

Ronald Reagan president and AIDS came along. The party came to a crashing end.

Eventually, I found out that I was negative and my closest friends were also negative, although some of them didn't remain negative. I remember there was one summer—I believe it was '87—there were 7 weeks when there was at least one funeral per week.

Then, of course, after they figured out what caused AIDS, I made every attempt to have protected sex. I was a top, so I assume, in retrospect, that's what probably kept me from getting AIDS in the first place.

I certainly did have sexual relations with a number of people who later became ill. Back in those days, before we found out what was causing AIDS, nobody wore condoms. I mean, it was just ridiculous. If you got syphilis or gonorrhea, which I and my friends did, you just went and got an antibiotic. I had hepatitis A and B. I didn't get very sick; I got over it. Some of my friends got very sick; we all got hepatitis at the same time. I had a very close friend who died of hepatitis B in 2004. He got cirrhosis of the liver, then he got cancer of the liver; he was 71. I can only say I was lucky.

In the late '90s, my best friend, my lover, my partner at that time, we became, as years went by, a two-some. We no longer lived with others, although we were still both free to have sexual relations with other people, and we did. Now neither one of us does much of anything, frankly. He and I are like brothers now. He and I have lived together for 33 years.

I've always had other friends, but my main friend was the person who died of hepatitis B in 2004. I've missed the man greatly. He and I were not sexually involved at any point along the way, but we did share a lot of things. He was, outside of my partner, my best friend. I miss him greatly. He had such a wonderful sense of humor; right up to the end, he was making jokes. I would take him to the hospital, pick him up from the hospital or doctor, and he'd be making jokes.

I have always had people that I could confide in, other than my partner. There always have been at least a few friends. They change over the years. Some moved away; a lot of them died back in the '80s and even into the '90s, until they got the drugs to help them out.

My health is basically fine. I'm still negative as far as HIV is concerned, although there have been some problems. Back in 2001, when I retired, I became a victim of heat exhaustion, to the point that I kept fainting. I couldn't figure out why I was doing it, but later on I realized I was becoming dehydrated. The last time I passed out I had a terrible experience. I thought I was dying. I had seizures and my partner picked me up at the beach and got me in the car, but I was going out. I thought I was going to go out and not come back, but eventually it did stop. I have gotten over that, and I have to be careful on hot days. If I'm going out on my bike, I drink a ton of water all along the way, I go slow, or I just don't it at all.

I have recurring staph infections in my right leg. I've had them over the last number of years, and twice I landed in the emergency room, where they gave me intravenous antibiotics. The next-to-the-last time that happened was in January, and I got over that one, but in early April I got another staph infection. It's always the right foot. I got another staph infection and this time the antibiotic did not help, so they put me in the hospital. I was in the hospital for the better part of the week and they determined that I had

MRSA [methicillin-resistant *Staphylococcus aureus*], which is a multiple-resistant staph. There are very few antibiotics left that are effective against it. They started treatment in the hospital and they saw that it was working. The swelling in my leg went down. They sent me home, but they had to send out home healthcare nurses to teach me how to do the intravenous therapy. I had to do it twice a day for 4 weeks.

People can get staph infections from going to the gym. I can't say for sure, and I've discussed it with the doctors (I won't name the gym I went to), but in the last number of years, up until April, I would go to the steam baths, and I believe I must have picked up those staph infections there. So, I decided that it was time for me to stop. I was thinking I probably shouldn't be spending so much time on that anyway. It really wasn't that productive. The attendance in the baths had dropped since they passed the antismoking policy. Now I have a very good reason to stay away from places like that, and I don't miss it.

I'm retired. I'm relatively well off, but not rich. I don't have to worry about financial things. I can read as much as I want; I've always been a reader. I can use my mind. I also have attempted, over the years, to write novels. I have written a bunch of them, but they were always rejected. It's difficult to publish. I would always write about gay things, and that was always a difficult thing to do anyway. I've kept myself busy during my retirement: writing, and someday I might publish. I've written a series of four novels that are connected. The characters are prehistoric gay people. It isn't just the gay thing. It has to do a lot with religion and technological changes; there's farming, using and domesticating horses, and stuff like that.

The least-satisfying thing in my life, obviously, was AIDS and the destruction of so many human beings. Now the thing that concerns me most is my sister. She is three years older than me and she's got multiple sclerosis.

You don't expect your contemporaries to die. You expect you mother and father to die at some point. My parents lived long lives and they both died at home. They didn't have to go to a nursing home.

My friend, my partner, has developed, in the last several years, a mental illness. It's depression, but it's more than that. He spends most of his life in bed and he's ruining his physical health by being so inactive. It pains me to see it. At this point I do have to be a caretaker. I have to dole out his medicine every day because he gets confused taking his medicine. He takes too much of things, and he has had periods when he passes out. It's not a burden to take care of him, but I do know that, from now on, I am going to have to take care of him. Taking care of him is not a burden; I don't mind it. When you grow older, if you grow older with somebody, you very well might have to take care of that person. That's accepted. I lived with him for 33 years and I'm going to make sure that—whatever happens to him—he is in the best situation possible, given his mental thing. I feel so sorry for him, that he has to go through this. That's what bothers me more than anything. At first, when it was first coming on a number of years ago, you have a tendency to blame the person and think that they are just being nasty, but it isn't that. I can't blame him; I just have to accept that this is happening.

THE PRAXIS OF QUEER GERONTOLOGY

> I know—and the face knows—that I am no longer a "boy." I appear Young, yes—but, inside, it's as if miles of years have stretched since I left that window in El Paso.
>
> —RECHY *(2013 [1963], p. 803)*

I BEGAN THIS JOURNEY WONDERING about the experiences of older gay men living with HIV. The route has been tortuous. I reversed, turned, deleted, hesitated, and even questioned the destination. I began by seeing the aging of gay men with HIV as a new chapter of the epidemic. Soon I realized I needed to broaden the view to the aging of gay men, regardless of HIV status. The lives of these men with HIV take place within the spheres of sexuality and identity, and, conversely, the aging of the Gayby Boomers is most certainly marked by HIV, if not in a personal, biomedical sense, definitely culturally, socially, and politically.

The Baby Boomer generation is arriving at old age, and a new phenomenon is being created: older LGBT people. As the world watched marriage equality being realized in the United States, I saw a danger in that visibility: the privileging and normalizing of certain identities and relationships at the exclusion of others, the queer—the "undignifying" quarters of ourselves and our communities. We were granting acceptance and dignity to some, while pointing at the shame of the weak, the lonely, the addict, the hustler, and the persons of color. I found, in the lives of the Gayby Boomers to whom I talked, a struggle to create a life caused by the clashes between their own sense of self and the social and cultural demands of the prevailing gay and old age worlds. Because they are assigned the labels of "older gay men" and "seniors," they encounter the task, again, of making sense of themselves and their friendships and their connections with others in a context ruled by norms that do not suit them. I came to see old age and gerontology as a robust bastion of heterosexuality, medicine, and our market economy.

My first readings on the topic, although informative, were boring. They came from public health and gerontology. They reduce old age, bodies, HIV, and sexuality to a set of "conditions" to be treated. They ignore the other side of aging—the human and social perspective; the intersections of race, social class, and sexuality. They promote "successful aging"—an idea now widely established in state policies, LGBT organizations, and in our psyche. When I juxtaposed the notion of successful aging with the experiences of the men I met, I learned that, although bringing some dignity to old age, the ethics of aging successfully shames queers (e.g., sexual deviants) and fat, lazy, alcoholic, and lonely older people. Some of the men I interviewed embrace this ethic to make themselves respectable and esteemed; yet they, themselves, and others cannot—and do not—want to abide by that script.

I also appreciated the insights and the limits of queer and sexuality theories. In the stories of Gayby Boomers, we see that the identities of "gay," "black," "HIV positive," and "older LGBT," for instance, do not capture their lives fully.

These identities are unstable, fractured, and, at times, missing. We also see that men, in an effort to make sense of old age, attempt to form bonds with others and recreate what they practiced in their youth: connections with other men outside social institutions and norms. But, queer theory still falls short in dealing with the material aspects of the self: the uneven distribution of resources required for daily living and its linkages with sexuality, race, and age.

And, unexpectedly, the journey has taken me back to a place I visited in my book *Compañeros* (Ramirez-Valles, 2011). There, I spoke about the solidarity (*compañerismo*) among Latin American gay men as the means by which they invent their place in the larger society, and confront whiteness and heterosexuality. I argued that this type of association could not exist in the U.S. individualistic and white gay world, and that it is very difficult for white men to join Latinos because of the racial structures with which we live. I have not changed my point of view, but I find some of the same qualities of *compañerismo* through the course of the narrated lives of Gayby Boomers. This is evident in two historical moments: the gay liberation movement and the AIDS epidemic.

The stories of aging the men shared with me cannot be explained in a single, all-encompassing theory or statement. Notions such as identity construction, queer, sexuality, historical change, transitions, embodiment, medicalization, social class, race, and intersections certainly help us both situate the aging of gay men and interpret their subjective experiences. But, they are not sufficient. And it is not my intention to provide a sweeping explanation of their narratives, because it has not been my interest to psychoanalyze or microdissect their stories. Yet, the individual and collective voices offer critical insights to the praxis of queer gerontology. Here I offer what I have learned about gay men's perspectives on aging and propose ways to transform gerontology. More than submitting an agenda or a prescription, I present reflections, pointers, and interrogations.

I focus on three joined themes: identity, shame, and the friendships and associations of gay men. I rely on a couple of scholars who write on queer sociology, primarily Michael Warner (1999), and the work of Michel Foucault (1997, 1998). Although these two scholars deal with aging and race only tangentially (and, yes, dismiss social class systems), their critique of identity and their analysis of shame and queer connections—"friendships" and "horizontal conjunctions" in Foucault's terms—are useful in reading gay men's stories of aging and constructing queer gerontology.

In examining the preceding stories, we see that the lives of these men, and the course they have taken, cannot be condensed to sex and sexuality. Through the course of their being, men's sexual desires and practices did have an influence, but were not the only forces—and perhaps not the most powerful—in shaping who they are. Their identities are not firm or uniform; they are fragmented across time and at any given moment. In particular, they escape the binaries of homosexual–heterosexual and old–young. They are queer, in the manner outlined by Valocchi (2005): "individual desires, practices, and affiliations cannot be accurately defined by the sex of object choice" (p. 754). They are also affected by racial, ethnic, age, and social class systems. For some men, still, the critical elements in their lives came from social and political events such as the antiwar and civil rights movements and AIDS. Then, in the same way that the meaning of old age in the United States is variable (Cronin & King,

2010)—unlike what mainstream gerontology and policies for the old portray—we find various connotations of old age among gay men.

Although some of the accounts of the men speak clearly to our institutionalized scripts about gay and old age, others depart. Different from what queer theorists would lead us to think, however, I find a robust accent on social class location, and this coincides frequently with racial and HIV status. Access to material and cultural resources—for everyday life and to make sense of one's self—is established early in life by social class position and is difficult to undo, even more so in older age.

Warner (1999) reminds us, nonetheless, that identity and shame are tied together. Shame is in the creation of queer experience, as it is at the core of AIDS. It runs through men's narratives. There is shame in the homosexual desire, in nonmonogamous and casual sex, "unprotected sex," and in the impulsive sex act. Much of the work of the contemporary and post-AIDS LGBT movement has been centered on identities (e.g., gay men, lesbian, transgender) in an effort to destigmatize and, in Warner's view, achieve respectability. These identities are professed as free of shame, as when gay men claim, "Sex does not define me," "Sex is only one part of me," and when they join the institution of marriage, vowing faithfulness and monogamy. But this move is at the expense of the queer, the other. We shame the "cheating" husbands, the single and lonely gay men, the hustler, and the polyamorous. But shame is not gone and Warner urges us to embrace it, not to treat it, but to experience freedom.

In shame I find a confluence between queer and aging. We shame the weak, unkempt, and uncontrollable old self as we shame the queer. The female aging body, a strand of feminist scholarship argues, is the target of shame (Twigg, 2004). We also see this reflected in gay men's work on the body as a way to deflect the shame brought up by AIDS. The ethics of successful aging, as the current LGBT movement, attempts to erase the shame to bring respectability. We should not confuse the present-day emphasis on sex—gay or straight "healthy sex life"—in old age as a sign of deshaming. Rather, sex is being constrained further to the field of medicine and psychology, and the privacy of our bedrooms, incited by the interests of pharmaceutical companies.

One of the dangers of successful aging is that it is an individual, private ethic. Warner (1999) cautions us that the isolation and privatization of our lives creates the context for shame. In such conditions, we have limited or no access to other knowledge, practices, and ways of being to make sense of ourselves and to recognize and communicate our shame. The implication is that only in solidarity and the open circulation of various forms of being we may replace shame fully with dignity (Warner, 1999).

In camaraderie, gay men realize and accept shame. It is in the margins of institutions that they are able to create, via their same-sex desire, alternative scripts. This is what Warner (1999) refers to the "queer ethics," which echo's Foucault's (1997) proposition that, in the relationships men create, friendships and horizontal conjunctions, through their homosexual desires, lies the promise to escape and confront power (Myers, 2008). I pose, then, that these connections are central in queer gerontology. Although I see shades of romanticism in both Foucault's and Warner's trust in gay men's relations, the notion is relevant in thinking about alternative ways of aging.

The stories of *Queer Aging* are infused with the creative bonds men build with other men through their sexual desire: friendships, friends with benefits, sex with strangers, casual sex—and its contemporary version: NSA (no-strings-attached), open relationships and *ménages à trois*. These forms of relating to one another are outside the norms of heterosexually, marriage, family, and the market economy. These bonds are fluid, contextual, and, by their nature, fragile. They have norms, but they are different from those of heterosexual institutions. Against the background of marriage and coupledom, gay men, like some of the men here, show that intimacy, love, sex, friendship, casual sexual encounters, and group sex are not opposite; they all can coexist (Warner 1999).

"Sex drive and passion die with the longevity of the relationship. People change; the relationship changes," my friend Andy said to me about this life with Owen (not their actual names). His confidences offer a pointed illustration. Andy and Owen have been together for 15 years. Both are in their late 50s and live a comfortable middle-class life. And both of them use Grindr, but separately. Andy uses the app for casual sex and conversation. His profile shows his handsome face but does not state his age or the fact that he is partnered. He tells me that after a few years of being a couple, they decided to open their sexual life. "The impulse to have sex ceases." Years ago they confronted the lack of passion and agreed to pursue sexual encounters freely. The idea of inviting others to have sex with them, as in a *ménage à trois*, was not on the table. Owen was not interested. He had a previous relationship, which lasted almost a decade, in which the partner enjoyed threesomes and he felt obligated to take part for the sake of the relationship. Andy and Owen don't talk about their sexual affairs.

Andy says that Owen offers him support, companionship, and connections with others. They do not live together. Each of them has his own home, to which they feel attached for a variety of reasons. They spend half of the week together—from Thursday to Sunday—in Andy's home. Yet, jointly they own a property in a resort community close to the water, where they live most of the summer. They profess commitment to one another but have no intention of marrying. As he tells me about his Grindr encounters, Andy states, "We all are in the same boat, but heterosexual couples pretend they are happy. They are boring. Their lives, if you look into them, are a mess. Monogamy is an invention, a lie; we all know that."

My friend's account is not exclusive of a white and middle-class temperament. These types of agreements, outside institutions, exist across social status (Heaphy, 2007). They are not always created by choice, explicitly made, or free of their own conflicts. Yet, the point is that these arrangements reject the constraints of heterosexuality and acknowledge instability, experimentation, and mutability in our sexual lives (Heaphy, 2007). These diverse liaisons may, at times, fuse to create a political force (in our popular use of the term) such in the gay liberation and AIDS movements (Cohen, 1999; Gould, 2009; Stockdill, 2003).

These friendships, horizontal conjunctions, or sometimes called "associative practices" (Myers, 2008) run through the life course and may provide the context for the exercise of freedom. Scholars in the life course field, such as Elder (1994), speak about our affiliations with others in terms of "interdependence," yet with a clear focus on normative relations. The concept of friendship in Foucault's work (1997) is qualitatively different from our common daily usage. He underscores liaisons formed beyond or in the periphery of gender and heterosexuality, and their related institutions of marriage, schools, religion, and economy. Friendship is what makes homosexuality a creative force, not the same-sex act in and of itself, or our gay identity, because it connects us, allowing us to communicate, circulate alternative ways of being, and deprivatize our existence (Foucault, 1997; Kingston. 2009; Myers, 2008). It also may foster autonomy, unlike, say, marriage and religious groups. The meaning of autonomy here is different from the one traditional gerontologists use: control and independence. It refers to the praxis of self-reflection and the making of novel forms of being. The task of creating one's self continually in opposition to normative structures and in reflexivity takes place precisely in our associations with others (Wong, 2013). Unlike political and social movements, the purpose of these connections is not to seize power, but to evade normalization—the gaze of power, in Foucault's terms (Wong, 2013).

Again, I'm not referring either to the very popular social support groups, as they are dominated by psychology and social work. Still, I have observed instances in which these traditional relational settings lead inadvertently to friendships among gay (and older gay) men. In one of the "senior LGBT" groups I attended, a smaller group of men, who were strangers before, would meet in their homes to hang out and have sex. Prime Timers, likewise, is a very traditional volunteer association, but on a very few occasions, I have witnessed cross-generational relations and the formation of liaisons of older gay men outside the organizations' rituals. In another project, I learned that gay men in recovery groups, such as drúg or sex addicts anonymous, on occasion create bonds that cross gender and sexual orientation outside the norms of the therapeutic script, and experiment with ways of making sense of themselves as "addicts" in recovery.

Recently outed by the *New York Times* (Halberstadt, 2015), the commune of queers or "LGBTQ nonconformist" is another illustration of horizontal junctures. Inspired by the Radical Faeries movement, people—many of them of older age—have created small, isolated communities countering the LGBT movement and heteronormativity. They resist assimilation and visibility, for example, by opposing any presence on the Internet. The groups develop their own set of rules of coexistence in a democratic process and rely on learned local and indigenous ways.

The LGBT movement, including its new "seniors" addition, is working against associate practices by promoting rights and inclusion into social institutions. Disremembering and the generational disruptions annihilate their continuity further. For example, LGBT organizations and SAGE have invested efforts in creating LGBT-friendly housing for seniors across the country. Many of these housing developments are a partnership among governments, not-for-profit organizations, and LGBT agencies. They are situated in LGBT neighborhoods and include both LGBT and heterosexual residents (of course, by law, they cannot discriminate on the basis of sexual orientation). This structure of living in retirement, however, rests on the idea of identity and gay–straight, young–old, single–couple entrenched dichotomies (Laws, 1994), hindering associate practices.

Furthermore, the systems of race and social class make it difficult to consider the horizontal conjunctures as a viable alternative in queer gerontology. As I have argued before (Ramirez-Valles, 2011), in the U.S. context, alliances between white gay men and gay men of color are mired in fear, resentment, shame, and stigma. This is why I am cautious about the queer promise of Warner (1999) and the horizontal junctures of Foucault (1997).

Throughout my participation in senior LGBT organizations, groups, and events, I witness the invisibility of older people of color. Blacks, Latinos, Asian Americans, and Native Americans, apparently, do not age or reach old age. I am exaggerating a little, because there some rare exceptions (Lashomb, 2015). On occasion, I would see a couple of black women and perhaps one black man. That's all. During my research, I attended a reception to announce the launching of a major national program for senior LGBT people. I, not yet an older person, was the only person of color in the room. And nobody raises the issue or questions it. That is the status quo and the invisibility of large sectors of our society.

I had a similar experience in the meetings at the American Society on Aging (ASA). The LGBT Aging Issues Network, a group within ASA, promotes actively the visibility of older queer people through workshops, panels, and meetings. Their work is admirable, because the LGBT Aging Issues Network works at the margins of the larger ASA. Yet, this group rarely speaks out on race and HIV. Black and Latino folks are nearly absent.

I am not making LGBT organizations solely responsible for this. There are a few individuals in those agencies concerned about the lack of color in their membership. This is a reality some of us in academic circles and community organizations are dealing with and trying to figure out. The point, as I hope I have shown, is not to argue for visibility and inclusion, but to acknowledge the limits of those spaces and agendas. They emerge from a very limited, privileged, and localized position, presuming they speak for all. The centralization of the older LGBT phenomenon in a few (state-supported) agencies is dangerous, and that is why I believe we need to turn our attention to the horizontal connections older gay men are crafting.

"What relationships, through homosexuality, can be established, invented, multiplied, and modulated?" (Foucault, 1997, p. 135). This is what Foucault invites us to think in the praxis of queer life. Our gay ethic, he goes on to say, "is not to identify with the psychological traits and the visible masks of the homosexual, but to try to define and develop a way of life" (p. 138). There is a new policing confronting gay men; we may call it age or aging. After the gay liberation movement, AIDS, and LGBT rights, the question posed at the beginning of this paragraph thus becomes relevant again.

In contemporary literature and popular media, older gay authors offer two contrasting explorations to the aging question (Weinstein, 2007). One takes the pop-psychology route: visibility, acceptance, recognition, healthy sex life. The other relies on the remembering of the gay liberation movement and AIDS, giving us a gloomy view. But both show that aging gay men are dealing with losing sex appeal, the grief of AIDS, melancholia of a better and happier life behind, and the loneliness that comes with age in general.

The answers and the transformation of gerontology will not be on a large scale. They will not mirror the wide strokes of previous movements or the sweeping disciplinary changes marked by gender and ethnic studies, for example. They are being worked out in small spaces and subjectivities.

Our aim should not be to set an across-the-board agenda, but to foster the creation of multiple types knowledge and autonomous contexts.

What ways of being could we create now to escape the policing of age, identity, medicine, heterosexuality, and the market? We must insist on asking this question.

REFERENCES

Cohen, C. J. (1999). *The boundaries of blackness: AIDS and the breakdown of black politics*. Chicago, IL: University of Chicago Press.

Cronin, A., & King, A. (2010). Power, inequality and identification: Exploring diversity and intersectionality amongst older LGB adults. *Sociology*, *44*(5), 876–892.

Elder, H. G. (1994). Time, human agency, and social change perspectives on life course. *Social Psychology Quarterly*, *57*, 4–15.

Foucault, M. (1997). Friendship as a way of life. In Paul Rabinow (Ed.), *Ethics and truth* (pp. 135–140). New York, NY: New Press.

Foucault, M. (1998). Technologies of the Self. In Paul Rabinow (Ed), *Ethics: Subjectivity and Truth Essential Works of Foucault, 1954–1984, Vol. 1* (pp. 223–251). New York, N Y: The New Press.

Gould, D. (2009). *Moving politics: emotion and ACT UP's fight against AIDS*. Chicago, IL: University of Chicago Press.

Halberstadt, A. (2015, August 6). Out of the woods [Online]. *The New York Times Magazine*. Available: http://mobile.nytimes.com/2015/08/09/magazine/out-of-the-woods.html.

Heaphy, B. (2007). Sexualities, gender and ageing: Resources and social change. *Current Sociology*, *55*(2), 193–210.

Kingston, M. (2009). Subversive friendships: Foucault on homosexuality and social experimentation. *Foucault Studies*, *7*, 7–17.

Lashomb, N. (2015, September). *Invisible no more: LGBT elders of color come to the forefront* [Online]. Available: http://www.therainbowtimesmass.com/2015/09/03/invisible-no-more-lgbt-elders-of-color-come-to-the-forefront/.

Laws, G. (1994). Aging, contested meanings, and the built environment. *Environment and Planning, 26*(11), 1787–1802.
Myers, E. (2008). Resisting Foucauldian ethics: associative politics and the limits of the care of the self. *Contemporary Political Theory, 7*, 125–146.
Rechy, J. (2013 [1963]). *City of night*. New York, NY: Grove Press. [E-reader version].
Ramirez-Valles, J. (2011). *Compañeros: Latino activists in the face of AIDS*. Urbana-Champagne, IL: University of Illinois Press.
Stockdill, B. C. (2003). *Activism against AIDS: at the intersections of sexuality, race, gender, and class*. Boulder, CO: Lynne Rienner Publishers.
Twigg, J. (2004). The body, gender and age: Feminist insights in social gerontology. *Journal of Aging Studies, 18*, 59–73.
Valocchi, S. (2005). Not yet queer enough: The lessons of queer theory for the sociology of gender and sexuality. *Gender and Society, 19*(6), 750–770.
Warner, M. (1999). *The trouble with normal: Sex, politics, and the ethics of queer life*. New York, NY. The Free Press.
Weinstein, S. (2007). Fiction of desire. *Out, 16*(5), 50–53.
Wong, J. (2013). Self and others: the work of "care" in Foucault's care of the self. *Philosophy Today, 57*(1), 99–113.

INDEX

Note: An italic *f* following a page number indicates a figure.